LICHEN SCLEROSUS DIET COOKBOOK

Nourishing Recipes and Practical Guidance for Healing, Wellness, and Delicious Eating

Kingsley Klopp

To show our appreciation for your purchase, we're delighted to offer you these special bonuses as a heartfelt thank you

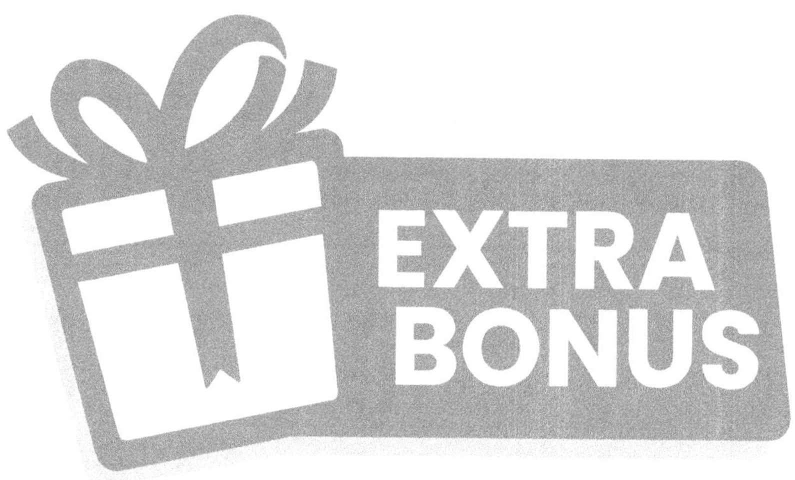

1. A Food Tracker Journal
2. Downloadable E-BOOK featuring full-color images of finished recipes

Table of Content

Important Note

We are delighted to present the **Lichen Sclerosus Diet Cookbook for Beginners,** a comprehensive guide filled with nourishing and delicious recipes designed to support your journey toward better health and well-being. As you explore the variety of meals we have carefully crafted, we want to share a few important considerations to ensure your experience is as beneficial and enjoyable as possible.

Firstly, it's essential to recognize that individual dietary needs and responses can vary significantly. What works wonders for one person might not be suitable for another. Therefore, we encourage you to listen to your body and adjust the recipes to fit your personal needs and preferences. Your comfort and health are paramount.

We highly recommend consulting with your healthcare provider or a registered dietitian, especially if you have any questions or concerns about the diet changes. They can provide personalized guidance tailored to your specific condition and overall health status, helping you make informed decisions that best support your journey with Lichen Sclerosus.

Additionally, please keep in mind that the nutritional information provided in this cookbook is approximate. Variations in ingredients, brands, and preparation methods can lead to differences in the final nutritional content of your meals. We strive to offer accurate and helpful data, but slight deviations are always possible.

Furthermore, If our cookbook has brought joy to your kitchen and table, we'd be thrilled to hear about your experiences in an Amazon review. On the flip side, if you stumble upon any hiccups while exploring our recipes, don't hesitate to get in touch at **kloppkingsley@gmail.com.** We're here to support your cooking journey every step of the

Our goal is to empower you with the knowledge and tools to create meals that not only nourish your body but also bring joy to your dining experience. We hope this cookbook serves as a valuable resource, inspiring you to explore new flavors and discover dishes that make you feel your best.

Thank you for entrusting us to be a part of your wellness journey. We wish you good health and happy cooking!

Introduction

Welcome to the **Lichen Sclerosus Diet Cookbook for Beginners!** If you've picked up this book, it's likely that you or someone you care about is navigating the challenges of Lichen Sclerosus (LS). Managing this chronic skin condition can feel overwhelming, but here's the silver lining: there's a powerful tool right at your fingertips—your diet. This cookbook is designed to be your guide, your companion, and your source of inspiration on the journey to managing LS through the healing power of food. Imagine starting your day with a breakfast that not only energizes you but also actively supports your body in reducing inflammation. Picture enjoying meals that are not just tasty but crafted with ingredients that help soothe your symptoms and promote overall well-being. This isn't a distant dream; it's a reality that you can achieve with the right knowledge and a bit of culinary creativity. And that's exactly what this book is here to provide.

Lichen Sclerosus is more than just a skin condition—it's a chronic inflammatory disease. Inflammation is a natural part of your body's defense system, but when it becomes chronic, it can cause persistent health issues. This is where an anti-inflammatory diet comes into play. By choosing foods that help reduce inflammation and avoiding those that trigger it, you can significantly improve your quality of life. This cookbook will show you how to make these choices with confidence and ease. Starting a new diet can be daunting, especially when you're already dealing with a challenging health condition. But don't worry, you're not alone on this journey. This cookbook is packed with information to help you understand the principles of an anti-inflammatory diet and how it specifically benefits those with Lichen Sclerosus. You'll learn about the foods that can help you manage your symptoms and those you should steer clear of. More importantly, you'll find a wealth of delicious, easy-to-follow recipes that make healthy eating a pleasure rather than a chore. Every recipe in this book is designed to be both nutritious and satisfying. Whether you're looking for a quick breakfast to kickstart your day, a hearty lunch to keep you going, or a comforting dinner to wind down, you'll find plenty of options that fit your needs and taste preferences. These recipes are created with real, whole foods that nourish your body and support your journey towards better health. Changing your diet is a big step, and it can be challenging. That's why this cookbook also offers practical tips, motivational advice, and real-life stories from people who have successfully managed their LS through dietary changes. These stories and tips are here to inspire you, to show you that it's possible to live well with LS, and to remind you that every small step you take towards better health is a victory.

But food is just one part of the equation. Managing LS involves a holistic approach that includes stress management, regular exercise, and adequate sleep. This book will touch on these aspects as well, providing a comprehensive guide to improving your overall well-being. The goal is to help you create a lifestyle that supports your health in every way possible. By picking up this cookbook, you've already taken a significant step towards managing your Lichen Sclerosus and improving your quality of life. Food has an incredible power to heal, and with the right choices, you can use it to your advantage. We're excited to join you on this journey, to help you discover the joys of healthy eating, and to support you every step of the way.

So let's get started. Let's explore the wonderful world of anti-inflammatory foods, try new recipes, and, most importantly, let's make every meal a step towards better health. Welcome to the **Lichen Sclerosus Diet Cookbook for Beginners**. Here's to a future filled with delicious food, better health, and renewed hope.

Chapter 1: Understanding Lichen Sclerosus
What is Lichen Sclerosus?

Lichen Sclerosus (LS) is a condition that many may have never heard of, yet it silently impacts thousands of lives worldwide, predominantly women. This chronic skin disorder is more than just a medical term; it is a daily battle, an emotional journey, and a story of resilience and hope. To truly grasp the weight of LS, it's essential to discuss its origins, causes, development over time, and the profound impact it has on those who live with it.

Historical Context and Origins

Lichen Sclerosus, first described in medical literature in the late 19th century, derives its name from the Greek word "leichen" meaning tree moss and "sclerosus" meaning hard. This nomenclature reflects the appearance of the affected skin, which often becomes thickened and scar-like. Over the years, our understanding of LS has evolved, yet it remains a mysterious and often misunderstood condition.

Historically, LS was an enigma, with limited knowledge and few treatment options. Early medical practitioners were baffled by its presentation and progression. It was only through decades of observation, research, and patient experiences that a clearer picture began to emerge. Despite these advancements, LS still poses many questions, leaving patients and healthcare providers in search of answers.

The Causes: A Complex Puzzle

The precise cause of Lichen Sclerosus remains elusive, contributing to the frustration and emotional turmoil experienced by those affected. However, research has identified several potential factors that may contribute to its development:

1. Autoimmune Factors: One of the most widely accepted theories is that LS has an autoimmune component. In autoimmune diseases, the body's immune system mistakenly attacks its own tissues. This theory is supported by the observation that LS often occurs in individuals with other autoimmune conditions such as thyroid disease, vitiligo, and alopecia areata. However, the exact mechanism behind this autoimmune response remains a subject of ongoing research.

2. Genetic Predisposition: Genetics may also play a significant role in the development of LS. Studies have shown a familial tendency, suggesting that individuals with a family history of LS may be at higher risk of developing the condition. However, a direct genetic link has yet to be definitively established, and more research is needed to understand the hereditary aspects of LS.

3. Hormonal Influences: Hormonal changes, particularly a decrease in estrogen levels, are thought to influence the onset and progression of LS. This is why the condition is often seen in postmenopausal women, although it can affect women of all ages, as well as men and children. The role of hormones in LS is complex and not fully understood, but it underscores the multifaceted nature of the disease.

4. Environmental Triggers: External factors such as trauma or injury to the skin, infections, or certain medications may act as triggers for LS in susceptible individuals. The exact nature of these triggers and how they interact with the body to cause LS is not fully understood. Environmental factors, combined with genetic and autoimmune predispositions, create a complex puzzle that researchers are still striving to piece together.

Development Over Time

Lichen Sclerosus is a chronic condition, meaning it persists over a long period, often for life. Its progression can vary greatly among individuals, making each person's journey with LS unique. Understanding the typical progression of LS can provide insight into the challenges faced by those living with the condition.

Initial Stages

In the early stages, LS may present as small, white spots on the skin, which might go unnoticed or be mistaken for another skin issue. As the condition progresses, these spots can merge into larger patches, causing the skin to become thin, wrinkled, and fragile. This fragility can lead to tearing, bleeding, and significant discomfort.

Chronic Impact

As LS evolves, it can cause considerable physical and emotional distress. The skin can become so delicate that everyday activities, such as walking, sitting, or sexual intercourse, become painful. Scarring can lead to changes in the anatomy, particularly in the genital area, which can be both physically and emotionally devastating. Living with Lichen Sclerosus requires continuous management and adaptation. While there is no cure, various treatments can help control symptoms and prevent complications. Topical corticosteroids are the mainstay of treatment, helping to reduce inflammation and improve skin condition. Other therapies, including hormone replacement, immunosuppressants, and even surgery in severe cases, may also be necessary.

Symptoms and Diagnosis of Lichen Sclerosus

Symptoms of Lichen Sclerosus

Lichen Sclerosus manifests differently in each person, with symptoms ranging from mild to severe. The symptoms can develop gradually or appear suddenly and can vary based on the affected area. Here, we delve into the common symptoms, their progression, and the challenges they pose.

Common Symptoms

1. White Patches of Skin: One of the hallmark symptoms of LS is the appearance of white, patchy skin. These patches are often shiny and smooth and can be found on the genital and anal areas, though they may also occur on the upper body, breasts, and arms.
2. Skin Fragility: The affected skin often becomes thin and fragile, making it prone to tearing, bleeding, and bruising. This fragility can lead to discomfort and pain, particularly in areas subjected to friction or pressure.
3. Itching and Discomfort: Itching is a common symptom and can range from mild to severe. Persistent itching can lead to scratching, which further damages the delicate skin, exacerbating the condition.
4. Pain: Pain is another frequent symptom, particularly during activities that involve friction or stretching of the skin. This includes walking, sitting, urination, bowel movements, and sexual intercourse. For many, the pain can be debilitating and impact daily activities and intimate relationships.
5. Blisters and Ulcers: In some cases, LS can cause blisters and ulcers, which can be painful and slow to heal. These open sores increase the risk of infection, further complicating the condition.
6. Skin Thickening and Scarring: Over time, the affected areas can become thickened and scarred. This can lead to a distortion of the normal anatomy, particularly in the genital area, causing additional complications such as difficulty with urination or sexual dysfunction.

Gender and Age-Specific Symptoms

- Women: In women, LS typically affects the vulva and can cause severe itching, burning, and pain. The vulvar skin may become fused and narrowed, leading to pain during intercourse (dyspareunia) and difficulties with urination.
- Men: Men with LS often experience symptoms on the foreskin and glans of the penis. This can result in phimosis (tightening of the foreskin), painful erections, and difficulty with urination.

- Children: In children, LS can be particularly challenging to diagnose as it may be mistaken for other skin conditions or infections. Symptoms in children often include itching, soreness, and visible white patches, which can cause significant discomfort and distress.

Diagnosis of Lichen Sclerosus

Accurate diagnosis of LS is essential for effective management and treatment. Diagnosis typically involves a combination of clinical evaluation and diagnostic tests. Here's a closer look at the diagnostic process:

Clinical Evaluation

The initial step in diagnosing LS involves a thorough clinical evaluation by a healthcare provider. This includes:

1. Medical History: The healthcare provider will take a detailed medical history, including any symptoms, their duration, and their impact on daily life. They will also inquire about any other medical conditions, particularly autoimmune disorders, which are often associated with LS.
2. Physical Examination: A physical examination is crucial for identifying the characteristic signs of LS. The healthcare provider will carefully examine the affected areas, looking for the distinctive white patches, skin thinning, and any signs of scarring or thickening.

Diagnostic Tests

While clinical evaluation is often sufficient for diagnosing LS, additional tests may be necessary to confirm the diagnosis and rule out other conditions.

1. Skin Biopsy: A skin biopsy is the most definitive test for diagnosing LS. During this procedure, a small sample of the affected skin is removed and examined under a microscope. The biopsy can reveal the characteristic histopathological features of LS, such as thinning of the epidermis, loss of the rete ridges, and changes in the collagen in the dermis. The biopsy can also help exclude other conditions, such as infections or skin cancers.
2. Histopathological Examination: The skin biopsy is sent to a pathology lab where a histopathologist examines the sample. The presence of thickened, sclerotic dermis and inflammation is indicative of LS. This examination can provide valuable information about the severity and extent of the condition.
3. Differential Diagnosis: Because LS can mimic other conditions, such as lichen planus, vitiligo, or chronic dermatitis, a differential diagnosis is often necessary. The healthcare provider may order additional tests or refer the patient to a specialist, such as a dermatologist or gynecologist, to ensure an accurate diagnosis.

The Emotional and Psychological Impact of Diagnosis

Receiving a diagnosis of Lichen Sclerosus can be a profound and emotional experience. For many, it provides relief in understanding the cause of their symptoms, but it can also bring feelings of fear, anxiety, and uncertainty about the future. The chronic nature of LS, along with its potential complications, can be overwhelming. Patients often experience a range of emotions, from relief at finally having a diagnosis to anxiety about the chronic nature of the disease and its impact on their lives. It's essential for healthcare providers to offer not only medical treatment but also emotional support, helping patients navigate their journey with LS.

Chapter 2: Introduction to Anti-Inflammatory Diet

What is an Anti-Inflammatory Diet?

An anti-inflammatory diet is more than just a way of eating; it's a lifestyle choice aimed at reducing chronic inflammation, which is a contributing factor to many diseases and health conditions. This diet focuses on consuming foods that help minimize inflammation in the body while avoiding foods that can exacerbate it.

Understanding Inflammation

Before delving into the specifics of an anti-inflammatory diet, it's important to understand what inflammation is. Inflammation is a natural and necessary process that the body uses to fight off infections and heal injuries. When you cut your finger, for example, the body's inflammatory response helps protect the wound from infection and begins the healing process. This type of acute inflammation is beneficial and usually short-lived.

However, chronic inflammation is a different story. Unlike acute inflammation, chronic inflammation persists over time and can occur even when there is no immediate injury or infection to combat. This prolonged inflammatory response can damage tissues and organs, contributing to a range of health problems, including heart disease, diabetes, arthritis, and certain cancers.

Principles of an Anti-Inflammatory Diet

The anti-inflammatory diet is designed to combat chronic inflammation by emphasizing foods that are known to reduce inflammatory markers in the body. Here are the core principles of this dietary approach:

1. Emphasizing Whole Foods: Whole, unprocessed foods are the foundation of an anti-inflammatory diet. This includes fresh fruits and vegetables, whole grains, lean proteins, and healthy fats. These foods are rich in essential nutrients and antioxidants that support the body's natural anti-inflammatory processes.

2. Incorporating Healthy Fats: Healthy fats, particularly omega-3 fatty acids, play a crucial role in reducing inflammation. Sources of these fats include fatty fish (such as salmon, mackerel, and sardines), flaxseeds, chia seeds, walnuts, and hemp seeds. Extra virgin olive oil is also a staple in an anti-inflammatory diet due to its high content of monounsaturated fats and polyphenols.

3. Choosing Antioxidant-Rich Foods: Antioxidants help neutralize free radicals, which can cause oxidative stress and contribute to inflammation. Foods rich in antioxidants include berries (blueberries, strawberries, raspberries), dark leafy greens (spinach, kale), nuts, seeds, and brightly colored vegetables (bell peppers, carrots, beets).

4. Prioritizing Fiber: A diet high in fiber supports gut health, which is closely linked to inflammation. Whole grains (such as quinoa, brown rice, and oats), legumes (beans, lentils, chickpeas), fruits, and vegetables are excellent sources of dietary fiber.

5. Reducing Processed Foods and Sugars: Processed foods often contain refined sugars, unhealthy fats, and artificial additives that can promote inflammation. Minimizing the intake of sugary beverages, snacks, processed meats, and fast foods is essential for reducing chronic inflammation.

6. Spices and Herbs: Certain spices and herbs have potent anti-inflammatory properties. Turmeric, ginger, garlic, cinnamon, and green tea are known for their ability to reduce inflammation and should be included regularly in the diet.

Practical Application of an Anti-Inflammatory Diet

Implementing an anti-inflammatory diet involves making thoughtful food choices and establishing healthy eating habits. Here are some practical tips to get started:

1. Plan Your Meals: Meal planning can help ensure that you include a variety of anti-inflammatory foods in your diet. Prepare meals in advance to avoid relying on processed or fast foods.
2. Cook at Home: Home-cooked meals give you control over the ingredients and cooking methods, allowing you to prioritize whole foods and healthy fats. Experiment with new recipes and cooking techniques to keep your meals interesting and enjoyable.
3. Stay Hydrated: Drinking plenty of water is essential for overall health and can help reduce inflammation. Herbal teas, particularly green tea and turmeric tea, are also great options for their anti-inflammatory properties.
4. Listen to Your Body: Pay attention to how different foods make you feel. Some individuals may have specific food sensitivities or allergies that can trigger inflammation. Keeping a food diary can help identify and eliminate problematic foods from your diet.
5. Balance and Moderation: While it's important to focus on anti-inflammatory foods, it's also essential to maintain a balanced diet that includes a variety of nutrients. Moderation is key to sustainable healthy eating habits.

Benefits of an Anti-Inflammatory Diet for Lichen Sclerosus

Lichen Sclerosus (LS) is a chronic skin condition characterized by white, patchy skin that can become fragile and tear easily. This condition often affects the genital and anal areas, but it can appear on other parts of the body as well. While there is no cure for LS, managing the symptoms and preventing flare-ups are critical for improving the quality of life of those affected. One of the most effective ways to manage LS is through an anti-inflammatory diet. This dietary approach can offer several significant benefits for individuals living with Lichen Sclerosus.

Understanding the Role of Inflammation in Lichen Sclerosus

Lichen Sclerosus is believed to be influenced by chronic inflammation. Inflammation is the body's natural response to injury or infection, but when it becomes chronic, it can contribute to a range of health issues, including LS. The anti-inflammatory diet aims to reduce chronic inflammation, thereby alleviating symptoms and improving overall health.

Key Benefits of an Anti-Inflammatory Diet for Lichen Sclerosus

1. *Reduction of Chronic Inflammation*

The primary benefit of an anti-inflammatory diet for LS is the reduction of chronic inflammation. By consuming foods that have anti-inflammatory properties and avoiding those that promote inflammation, individuals can help calm the inflammatory response in their bodies. This can lead to a reduction in the symptoms of LS, such as itching, pain, and skin fragility.

2. *Improved Skin Health*

An anti-inflammatory diet is rich in nutrients that support skin health. Foods high in antioxidants, such as fruits and vegetables, help protect skin cells from damage and promote healing. Omega-3 fatty acids, found in fatty fish, flaxseeds, and walnuts, are known to improve skin elasticity and reduce inflammation, which can be particularly beneficial for individuals with LS.

3. *Enhanced Immune Function*

LS is thought to have an autoimmune component, meaning the immune system mistakenly attacks healthy tissue. An anti-inflammatory diet can help regulate the immune system, reducing the likelihood of autoimmune flare-ups. Nutrient-dense foods provide essential vitamins and minerals that support a balanced immune response, potentially decreasing the frequency and severity of LS symptoms.

4. *Gut Health Improvement*
The health of the gut microbiome plays a crucial role in managing inflammation throughout the body. An anti-inflammatory diet emphasizes fiber-rich foods, such as whole grains, legumes, fruits, and vegetables, which promote a healthy gut microbiome. A balanced gut microbiome can help reduce systemic inflammation and may improve symptoms of LS.

5. *Pain and Discomfort Management*
Chronic pain and discomfort are common symptoms of LS. By reducing inflammation, an anti-inflammatory diet can help alleviate pain and improve overall comfort. Foods such as turmeric and ginger have natural anti-inflammatory and analgesic properties, making them valuable additions to the diet of someone with LS.

6. *Weight Management*
Maintaining a healthy weight is important for managing LS, as excess weight can exacerbate inflammation. An anti-inflammatory diet, which focuses on whole, unprocessed foods, can help individuals achieve and maintain a healthy weight. This, in turn, can reduce the burden of inflammation on the body and help manage LS symptoms.

7. *Hormonal Balance*
Hormonal imbalances can influence the development and progression of LS. An anti-inflammatory diet helps stabilize blood sugar levels and supports overall hormonal health. Consuming a balanced diet with adequate healthy fats, proteins, and complex carbohydrates can help regulate hormones and reduce the risk of hormonal fluctuations that may trigger LS flare-ups.

8. *Improved Mental Health*
Chronic conditions like LS can take a toll on mental health, leading to feelings of anxiety and depression. An anti-inflammatory diet supports brain health by providing essential nutrients that promote cognitive function and emotional well-being. Foods rich in omega-3 fatty acids, antioxidants, and vitamins can help improve mood and reduce the psychological impact of living with a chronic condition.

Practical Application of an Anti-Inflammatory Diet for Lichen Sclerosus
To reap the benefits of an anti-inflammatory diet, individuals with LS should focus on incorporating the following foods into their daily meals:
- Fruits and Vegetables: Aim for a variety of colorful fruits and vegetables, which are high in antioxidants and essential vitamins.
- Healthy Fats: Include sources of omega-3 fatty acids such as fatty fish (salmon, mackerel, sardines), flaxseeds, chia seeds, and walnuts. Olive oil is another excellent source of healthy fats.

- Whole Grains: Choose whole grains like quinoa, brown rice, and oats over refined grains.
- Lean Proteins: Opt for lean proteins such as chicken, turkey, tofu, and legumes.
- Herbs and Spices: Use anti-inflammatory spices such as turmeric, ginger, garlic, and cinnamon in cooking.
- Nuts and Seeds: Incorporate a variety of nuts and seeds into snacks and meals.

Foods to Avoid and Foods to Include

Foods to Avoid for Lichen Sclerosus

Avoiding certain foods can help reduce inflammation and prevent exacerbating the symptoms of LS. Here are the key food groups and items to avoid:

1. Refined Sugars and Carbohydrates
   - Why to Avoid: Refined sugars and carbohydrates can cause spikes in blood sugar levels, leading to increased inflammation. High sugar intake can also weaken the immune system and contribute to overall health deterioration.
   - Examples: Sweets, candies, sugary beverages (sodas, energy drinks), white bread, pastries, and other baked goods made with refined flour.
2. Processed and Red Meats
   - Why to Avoid: Processed and red meats are high in saturated fats and can promote inflammation. They may also contain additives and preservatives that can trigger inflammatory responses.
   - Examples: Bacon, sausages, hot dogs, deli meats, beef, and lamb.
3. Dairy Products
   - Why to Avoid: Dairy products can be inflammatory for some people, particularly those who are lactose intolerant or have a sensitivity to casein, a protein found in milk.
   - Examples: Milk, cheese, butter, and ice cream.
4. Gluten
   - Why to Avoid: For individuals with gluten sensitivity or celiac disease, gluten can cause inflammation and exacerbate LS symptoms. Even for those without these conditions, reducing gluten intake can sometimes improve skin health.
   - Examples: Wheat, barley, rye, and products containing these grains (bread, pasta, cereals).
5. Alcohol
   - Why to Avoid: Alcohol can increase inflammation and irritate the skin. It can also interfere with the body's natural healing processes and weaken the immune system.
   - Examples: Beer, wine, spirits, and cocktails.
6. Trans Fats
   - Why to Avoid: Trans fats are highly inflammatory and can be found in many processed and fast foods. They contribute to systemic inflammation and can worsen LS symptoms.
   - Examples: Fried foods, margarine, commercially baked goods, and snacks with partially hydrogenated oils.

Foods to Include for Lichen Sclerosus

Including anti-inflammatory and nutrient-dense foods in your diet can help manage LS symptoms and promote overall health. Here are the key food groups and items to include:

1. Fruits and Vegetables
   - Why to Include: Fruits and vegetables are rich in antioxidants, vitamins, and minerals that support immune function and reduce inflammation. They provide essential nutrients that promote skin health and overall well-being.
   - Examples: Berries (blueberries, strawberries, raspberries), leafy greens (spinach, kale, arugula), cruciferous vegetables (broccoli, cauliflower, Brussels sprouts), and colorful vegetables (bell peppers, carrots, tomatoes).
2. Healthy Fats
   - Why to Include: Healthy fats, particularly omega-3 fatty acids, have strong anti-inflammatory properties. They support skin health, reduce inflammation, and improve immune function.
   - Examples: Fatty fish (salmon, mackerel, sardines), flaxseeds, chia seeds, walnuts, and extra virgin olive oil.
3. Whole Grains
   - Why to Include: Whole grains are a great source of fiber, which supports gut health and helps reduce inflammation. They also provide essential nutrients that contribute to overall health.
   - Examples: Quinoa, brown rice, oats, millet, and whole wheat (if not sensitive to gluten).
4. Lean Proteins
   - Why to Include: Lean proteins provide the necessary building blocks for tissue repair and immune function without contributing to inflammation. They help maintain muscle mass and overall strength.
   - Examples: Chicken, turkey, tofu, tempeh, beans, lentils, and legumes.
5. Nuts and Seeds
   - Why to Include: Nuts and seeds are packed with healthy fats, fiber, protein, and antioxidants. They help reduce inflammation and provide a satisfying, nutritious snack option.
   - Examples: Almonds, walnuts, sunflower seeds, and chia seeds.
6. Herbs and Spices
   - Why to Include: Certain herbs and spices have potent anti-inflammatory properties and can enhance the flavor of meals without the need for added salt or sugar.
   - Examples: Turmeric, ginger, garlic, cinnamon, and rosemary.
7. Fermented Foods
   - Why to Include: Fermented foods support gut health by providing beneficial probiotics. A healthy gut microbiome can reduce inflammation and improve overall health.
   - Examples: Yogurt (if tolerated), kefir, sauerkraut, kimchi, and kombucha.

Breakfast Recipes

1. Fruit and Nut Platter
Ingredients
- 1 cup mixed fresh berries (strawberries, blueberries, raspberries)
- 1 apple, sliced
- 1 pear, sliced
- 1 banana, sliced
- 1/2 cup almonds
- 1/2 cup walnuts
- 1/4 cup sunflower seeds
- 1/4 cup dried cranberries (unsweetened)

Instructions
1. Wash and prepare all the fresh fruits.
2. Arrange the mixed berries, apple slices, pear slices, and banana slices on a large platter.
3. Add almonds, walnuts, sunflower seeds, and dried cranberries to the platter.
4. Serve immediately and enjoy!

Nutrition Info per Serving
- Calories: 250
- Protein: 6g
- Fat: 12g
- Carbohydrates: 33g
- Fiber: 7g
- Sugar: 18g

Serves
4

Cooking Time
10 minutes

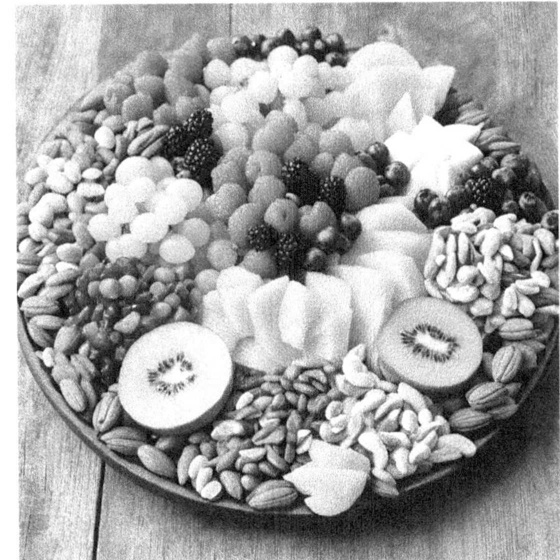

2. Polenta with Grilled Vegetables

Ingredients

- 1 cup polenta (cornmeal)
- 4 cups water
- 1 tablespoon olive oil
- 1 zucchini, sliced
- 1 red bell pepper, sliced
- 1 yellow bell pepper, sliced
- 1/2 cup cherry tomatoes, halved
- 1 tablespoon balsamic vinegar
- 1 teaspoon dried oregano
- 1/2 teaspoon garlic powder

Instructions

1. In a medium saucepan, bring water to a boil. Gradually whisk in the polenta and reduce heat to low.
2. Cook the polenta, stirring frequently, for about 20 minutes until thick and creamy. Remove from heat.
3. Preheat the grill to medium-high heat.
4. In a bowl, toss the zucchini, bell peppers, and cherry tomatoes with olive oil, balsamic vinegar, oregano, and garlic powder.
5. Grill the vegetables for about 5-7 minutes, until tender and slightly charred.
6. Serve the grilled vegetables over the polenta.

Nutrition Info per Serving

- Calories: 220
- Protein: 5g
- Fat: 7g
- Carbohydrates: 36g
- Fiber: 4g
- Sugar: 5g

Serves

4

Cooking Time

30 minutes

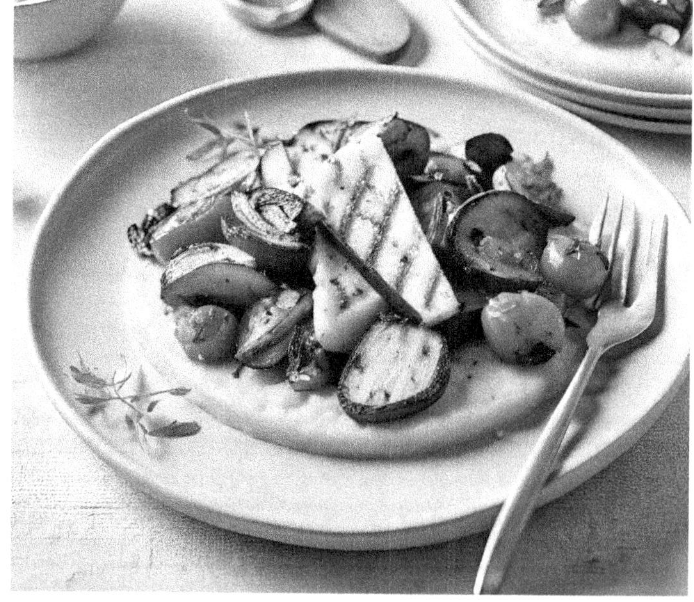

3. Kefir with Chopped Dates

Ingredients

- 2 cups plain kefir
- 1/2 cup dates, pitted and chopped
- 1/4 cup crushed walnuts
- 1 tablespoon honey (optional)

Instructions

1. Pour kefir into serving bowls.
2. Top with chopped dates and crushed walnuts.
3. Drizzle with honey if desired.
4. Serve immediately and enjoy!

Nutrition Info per Serving

- Calories: 180
- Protein: 7g
- Fat: 6g
- Carbohydrates: 27g
- Fiber: 3g
- Sugar: 18g

Serves
2

Cooking Time
5 minutes

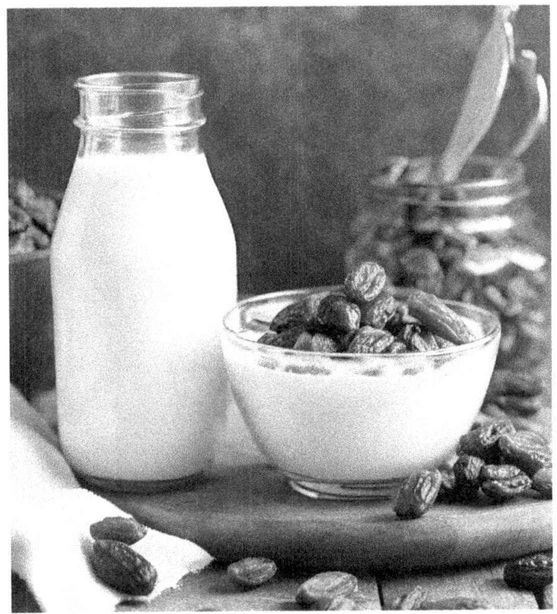

4. Apple Cinnamon Baked Oatmeal

Ingredients

- 2 cups rolled oats
- 2 teaspoons ground cinnamon
- 1 teaspoon baking powder
- 1/2 teaspoon ground nutmeg
- 2 cups almond milk (unsweetened)
- 1/4 cup maple syrup
- 1 large apple, peeled and diced
- 1 teaspoon vanilla extract
- 1/4 cup chopped pecans (optional)

Instructions

1. Preheat the oven to 375°F (190°C). Grease an 8x8-inch baking dish.
2. In a large bowl, mix the rolled oats, cinnamon, baking powder, and nutmeg.
3. Add the almond milk, maple syrup, diced apple, and vanilla extract to the bowl. Mix well.
4. Pour the mixture into the prepared baking dish and spread evenly.
5. Sprinkle the chopped pecans on top if using.
6. Bake for 35-40 minutes, until the oatmeal is set and lightly browned.
7. Let cool for a few minutes before serving.

Nutrition Info per Serving

- Calories: 220
- Protein: 5g
- Fat: 6g
- Carbohydrates: 38g
- Fiber: 5g
- Sugar: 12g

Serves

4

Cooking Time

45 minutes

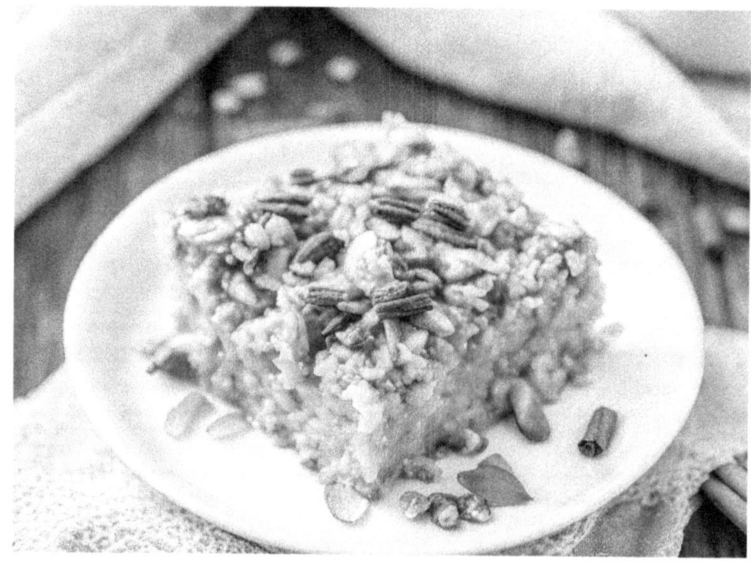

5. Savory Spinach Pancakes

Ingredients

- 1 cup fresh spinach leaves
- 1 cup chickpea flour (also known as gram flour or besan)
- 1/2 cup water
- 1/4 cup finely chopped onion
- 1/2 teaspoon garlic powder
- 1/2 teaspoon ground cumin
- 1/2 teaspoon turmeric powder
- 2 tablespoons olive oil for cooking

Instructions

1. In a blender, combine the spinach leaves and water. Blend until smooth.
2. In a mixing bowl, whisk together the chickpea flour, garlic powder, ground cumin, and turmeric powder.
3. Pour the spinach mixture into the dry ingredients and mix until well combined. The batter should be thick but pourable. Add more water if necessary.
4. Stir in the finely chopped onion.
5. Heat a tablespoon of olive oil in a non-stick skillet over medium heat.
6. Pour about 1/4 cup of the batter into the skillet, spreading it out into a pancake shape.
7. Cook for 2-3 minutes on each side until golden brown and cooked through.
8. Repeat with the remaining batter, adding more oil as needed.
9. Serve warm.

Nutrition Info per Serving

- Calories: 180
- Protein: 6g
- Fat: 10g
- Carbohydrates: 18g
- Fiber: 4g
- Sugar: 2g

Serves

4

Cooking Time

20 minutes

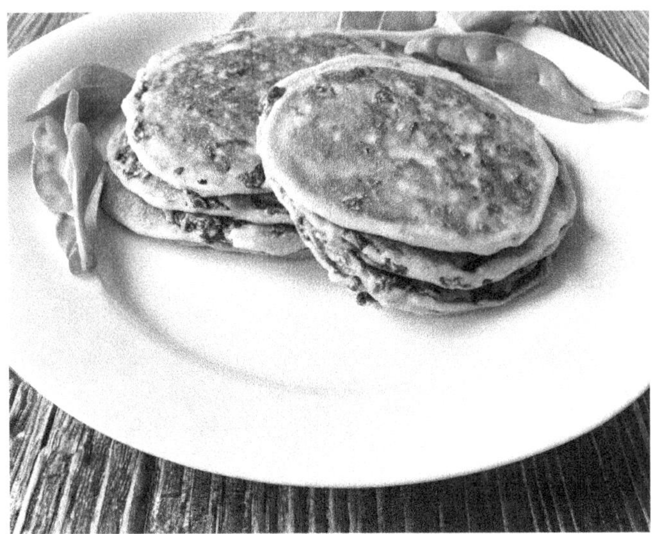

6. Nutty Porridge

Ingredients

- 1 cup rolled oats
- 2 cups almond milk (unsweetened)
- 1/4 cup chopped almonds
- 1/4 cup chopped walnuts
- 1 tablespoon chia seeds
- 1 tablespoon ground flaxseeds
- 1 tablespoon maple syrup
- 1 teaspoon ground cinnamon

Instructions

1. In a medium saucepan, combine the rolled oats and almond milk. Bring to a boil over medium heat.
2. Reduce heat to low and simmer for about 5-7 minutes, stirring occasionally, until the oats are tender and the porridge has thickened.
3. Stir in the chopped almonds, walnuts, chia seeds, ground flaxseeds, maple syrup, and ground cinnamon.
4. Cook for an additional 2 minutes, stirring to combine all ingredients evenly.
5. Serve warm.

Nutrition Info per Serving

- Calories: 250
- Protein: 7g
- Fat: 12g
- Carbohydrates: 30g
- Fiber: 6g
- Sugar: 7g

Serves

4

Cooking Time

15 minutes

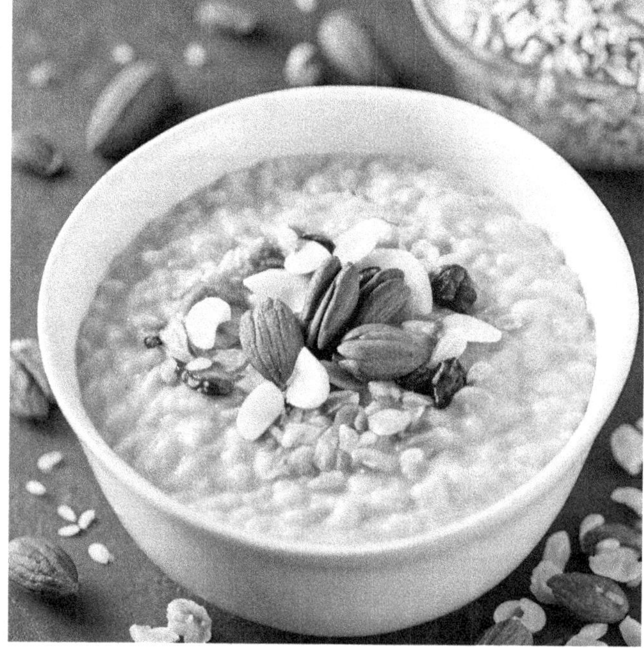

7. Beet and Carrot Juice

Ingredients

- 2 medium beets, peeled and chopped
- 4 medium carrots, peeled and chopped
- 1 apple, cored and chopped
- 1-inch piece of ginger, peeled
- 1 cup water

Instructions

1. In a blender or juicer, combine the beets, carrots, apple, ginger, and water.
2. Blend or juice until smooth.
3. If using a blender, strain the mixture through a fine mesh sieve or cheesecloth to remove the pulp.
4. Pour the juice into glasses and serve immediately.

Nutrition Info per Serving

- Calories: 120   Protein: 2g   Fat: 0g
- Carbohydrates: 29g   Fiber: 6g   Sugar: 18g

Serves 2

Cooking Time

10 minutes

8. Overnight Hemp Seeds

Ingredients

- 1/2 cup hemp seeds
- 1 cup almond milk (unsweetened)
- 1 tablespoon chia seeds
- 1 tablespoon maple syrup
- 1/2 teaspoon vanilla extract
- Fresh berries for topping (optional)

Instructions

1. In a jar or container, combine the hemp seeds, almond milk, chia seeds, maple syrup, and vanilla extract.
2. Stir well to combine.
3. Cover and refrigerate overnight.
4. In the morning, give the mixture a good stir. Add more almond milk if it's too thick.
5. Top with fresh berries if desired and serve.

Nutrition Info per Serving

- Calories: 220   Protein: 10g   Fat: 16g   Carbohydrates: 10g
- Fiber: 4g   Sugar: 6g

Serves 2

Cooking Time

5 minutes (plus overnight soaking)

9. Tempeh Bacon Lettuce Tomato Sandwich

Ingredients

- 8 ounces tempeh, thinly sliced
- 1/4 cup tamari or soy sauce
- 1 tablespoon maple syrup
- 1 teaspoon smoked paprika
- 1 tablespoon olive oil
- 4 slices whole grain bread
- 1 large tomato, sliced
- 4 leaves of lettuce
- 1 avocado, sliced

Instructions

1. In a bowl, combine the tamari, maple syrup, and smoked paprika. Add the sliced tempeh and marinate for at least 15 minutes.
2. Heat olive oil in a skillet over medium heat. Add the marinated tempeh slices and cook for 2-3 minutes on each side until crispy.
3. Toast the bread slices.
4. Assemble the sandwiches by layering the tempeh bacon, tomato slices, lettuce leaves, and avocado slices between two pieces of toast.
5. Serve immediately.

Nutrition Info per Serving

- Calories: 300
- Protein: 14g
- Fat: 18g
- Carbohydrates: 28g
- Fiber: 7g
- Sugar: 6g

Serves

2

Cooking Time

20 minutes

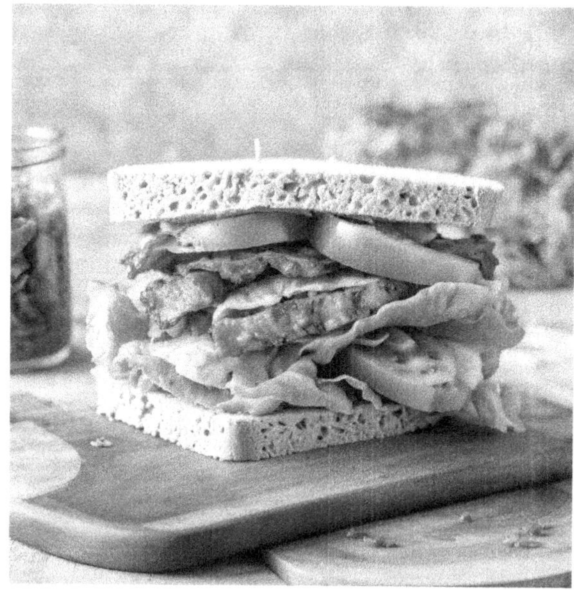

10. Flaxseed and Banana Muffins

Ingredients

- 1 cup almond flour
- 1/2 cup ground flaxseed
- 1/2 teaspoon baking soda
- 1 teaspoon ground cinnamon
- 2 ripe bananas, mashed
- 2 large eggs
- 1/4 cup honey
- 1 teaspoon vanilla extract
- 1/4 cup almond milk (unsweetened)

Instructions

1. Preheat the oven to 350°F (175°C). Line a muffin tin with paper liners.
2. In a large bowl, mix the almond flour, ground flaxseed, baking soda, and cinnamon.
3. In another bowl, combine the mashed bananas, eggs, honey, vanilla extract, and almond milk.
4. Pour the wet ingredients into the dry ingredients and mix until just combined.
5. Divide the batter evenly among the muffin cups.
6. Bake for 20-25 minutes, or until a toothpick inserted into the center comes out clean.
7. Let cool in the tin for 5 minutes before transferring to a wire rack to cool completely.

Nutrition Info per Serving

- Calories: 160
- Protein: 5g
- Fat: 9g
- Carbohydrates: 18g
- Fiber: 4g
- Sugar: 10g

Serves

12

Cooking Time

30 minutes

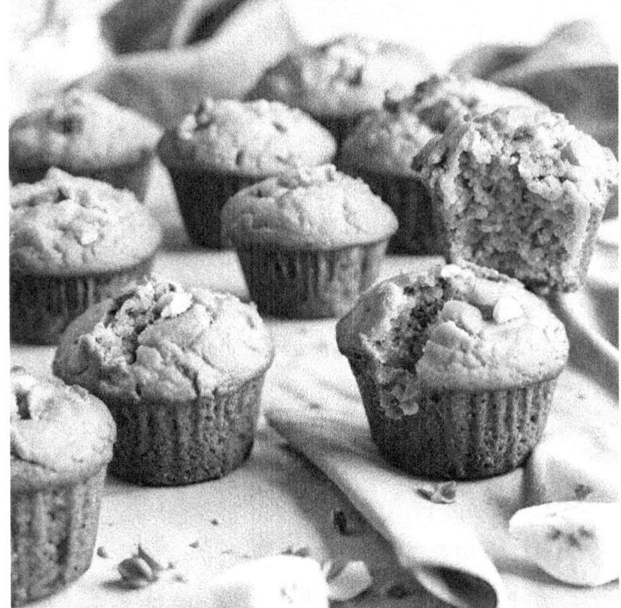

11. Sunflower Seed Butter on Gluten-Free Bread

Ingredients

- 4 slices gluten-free bread
- 1/2 cup sunflower seed butter
- 1 banana, sliced
- 1 tablespoon honey (optional)

Instructions

1. Toast the gluten-free bread slices.
2. Spread sunflower seed butter evenly on each slice.
3. Top with banana slices.
4. Drizzle with honey if desired.
5. Serve immediately.

Nutrition Info per Serving

- Calories: 250 Protein: 7g Fat: 15g
- Carbohydrates: 24g   Fiber: 4g   Sugar: 9g

Serves 4

Cooking Time

10 minutes

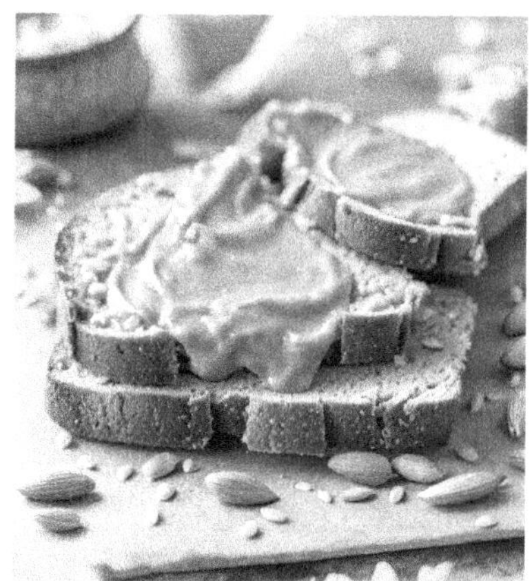

12. Herbal Tea with Rice Porridge

Ingredients

- 1 cup brown rice
- 4 cups water
- 1 cup almond milk (unsweetened)
- 1 tablespoon honey
- 1 teaspoon ground cinnamon
- 4 cups brewed herbal tea (such as chamomile or peppermint)

Instructions

1. In a medium saucepan, combine the brown rice and water. Bring to a boil, then reduce heat to low and simmer for 30-40 minutes, until the rice is tender.
2. Stir in the almond milk, honey, and ground cinnamon. Cook for an additional 5 minutes, until the porridge is creamy.
3. Serve the rice porridge hot with a cup of brewed herbal tea on the side.

Nutrition Info per Serving

- Calories: 180 Protein: 4g   Fat: 3g   Carbohydrates: 36g
- Fiber: 2g   Sugar: 6g

Serves 4

Cooking Time

45 minutes

13. Raspberry Coconut Porridge

Ingredients

- 1 cup rolled oats
- 2 cups coconut milk (unsweetened)
- 1/2 cup fresh or frozen raspberries
- 1 tablespoon chia seeds
- 1 tablespoon shredded coconut
- 1 tablespoon maple syrup

Instructions

1. In a medium saucepan, combine the rolled oats and coconut milk. Bring to a boil over medium heat.
2. Reduce heat to low and simmer for about 5-7 minutes, stirring occasionally, until the oats are tender and the porridge has thickened.
3. Stir in the chia seeds and maple syrup.
4. Serve topped with raspberries and shredded coconut.

Nutrition Info per Serving

- Calories: 220
- Protein: 5g
- Fat: 10g
- Carbohydrates: 28g
- Fiber: 6g
- Sugar: 8g

Serves

2

Cooking Time

10 minutes

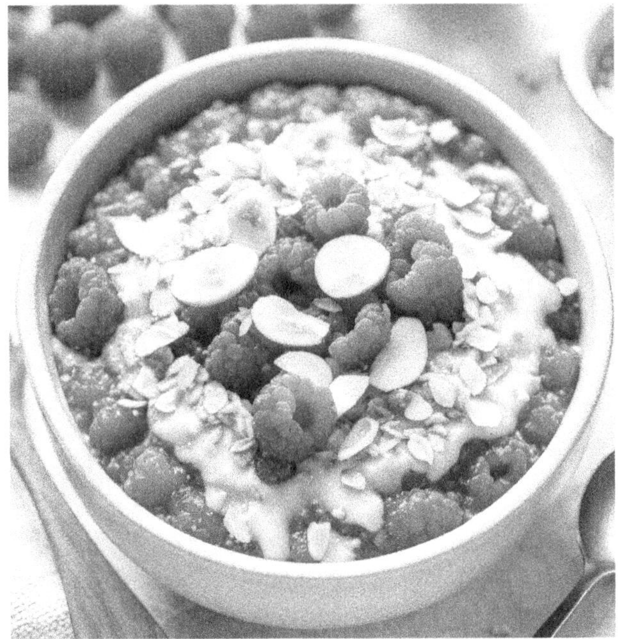

14. Spiced Lentil Breakfast Bowl

Ingredients

- 1 cup red lentils, rinsed
- 3 cups water
- 1 teaspoon ground turmeric
- 1 teaspoon ground cumin
- 1/2 teaspoon ground coriander
- 1 cup baby spinach
- 1/2 cup cherry tomatoes, halved
- 1 tablespoon olive oil
- 1 tablespoon lemon juice

Instructions

1. In a medium saucepan, combine the red lentils, water, turmeric, cumin, and coriander. Bring to a boil over medium-high heat.
2. Reduce heat to low and simmer for 15-20 minutes, until the lentils are tender and the water is absorbed.
3. Stir in the baby spinach and cook for an additional 2 minutes, until wilted.
4. Remove from heat and stir in the olive oil and lemon juice.
5. Serve in bowls topped with cherry tomatoes.

Nutrition Info per Serving

- Calories: 220
- Protein: 13g
- Fat: 6g
- Carbohydrates: 29g
- Fiber: 10g
- Sugar: 4g

Serves

2

Cooking Time

25 minutes

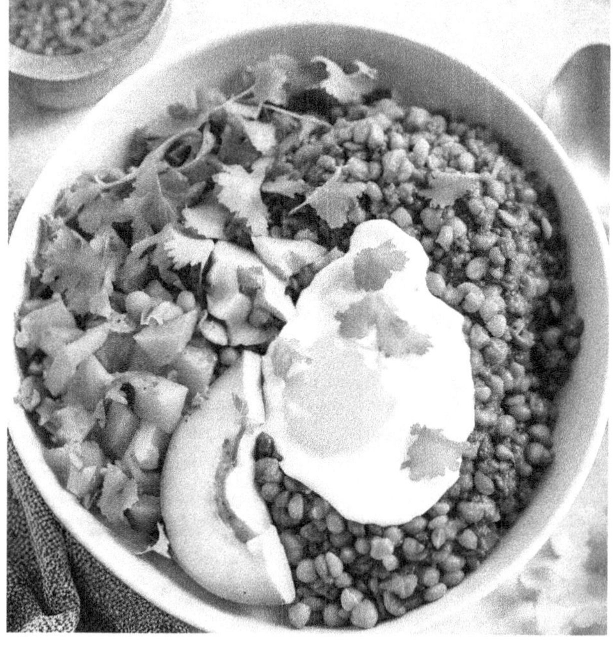

15. Cauliflower Breakfast Skillet

Ingredients

- 1 medium cauliflower, chopped into small florets
- 1 tablespoon olive oil
- 1 small onion, finely chopped
- 1 bell pepper, chopped
- 2 cloves garlic, minced
- 1 teaspoon turmeric powder
- 1/2 teaspoon cumin powder
- 1/2 teaspoon paprika
- 2 cups fresh spinach
- 4 large eggs
- 1 avocado, sliced (optional)

Instructions

1. Heat olive oil in a large skillet over medium heat.
2. Add the chopped onion and bell pepper, and sauté for about 5 minutes until softened.
3. Add the garlic, turmeric, cumin, and paprika, and cook for another 2 minutes.
4. Add the cauliflower florets and cook, stirring occasionally, for about 10 minutes until the cauliflower is tender.
5. Stir in the spinach and cook until wilted.
6. Create four small wells in the mixture and crack an egg into each well.
7. Cover the skillet and cook until the eggs are set to your liking, about 5 minutes.
8. Serve immediately, with sliced avocado on top if desired.

Nutrition Info per Serving

- Calories: 230
- Protein: 12g
- Fat: 14g
- Carbohydrates: 17g
- Fiber: 7g
- Sugar: 5g

Serves

4

Cooking Time

25 minutes

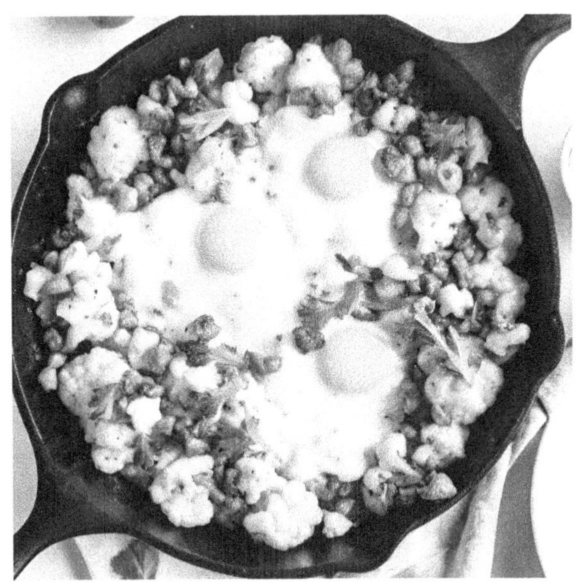

16. Zucchini Bread

Ingredients

- 1 1/2 cups almond flour
- 1/2 cup coconut flour
- 1 teaspoon baking soda
- 1 teaspoon ground cinnamon
- 1/2 teaspoon ground nutmeg
- 2 large eggs
- 1/4 cup honey
- 1/4 cup coconut oil, melted
- 1 teaspoon vanilla extract
- 1 1/2 cups grated zucchini

Instructions

1. Preheat the oven to 350°F (175°C). Grease a loaf pan or line it with parchment paper.
2. In a large bowl, combine almond flour, coconut flour, baking soda, cinnamon, and nutmeg.
3. In another bowl, whisk together the eggs, honey, melted coconut oil, and vanilla extract.
4. Pour the wet ingredients into the dry ingredients and mix until well combined.
5. Fold in the grated zucchini.
6. Pour the batter into the prepared loaf pan and smooth the top.
7. Bake for 45-50 minutes, or until a toothpick inserted into the center comes out clean.
8. Allow the bread to cool in the pan for 10 minutes before transferring to a wire rack to cool completely.

Nutrition Info per Serving

- Calories: 180
- Protein: 5g
- Fat: 12g
- Carbohydrates: 14g
- Fiber: 3g
- Sugar: 8g

Serves

8

Cooking Time

1 hour

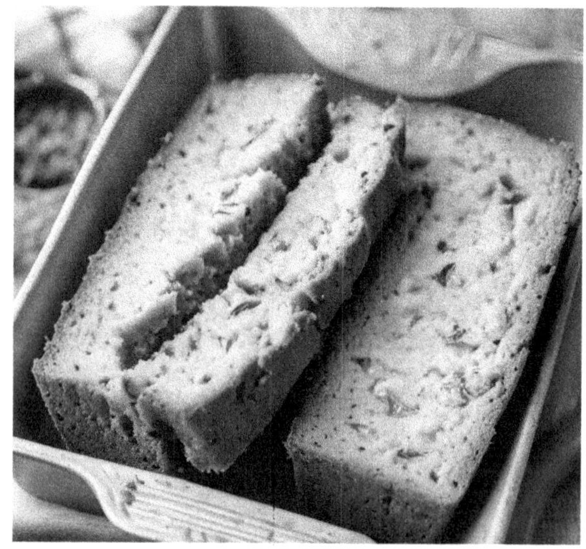

17. Berry and Kiwi Salad

Ingredients

- 1 cup strawberries, hulled and sliced
- 1 cup blueberries
- 1 cup raspberries
- 2 kiwis, peeled and sliced
- 1 tablespoon fresh lemon juice
- 1 tablespoon honey (optional)

Instructions

1. In a large bowl, combine the strawberries, blueberries, raspberries, and kiwi slices.
2. Drizzle with fresh lemon juice and honey if using.
3. Gently toss to combine.
4. Serve immediately.

Nutrition Info per Serving

- Calories: 90   Protein: 1g Fat: 0g   Carbohydrates: 22g
- Fiber: 5g Sugar: 14g

Serves 4

Cooking Time 10 minutes

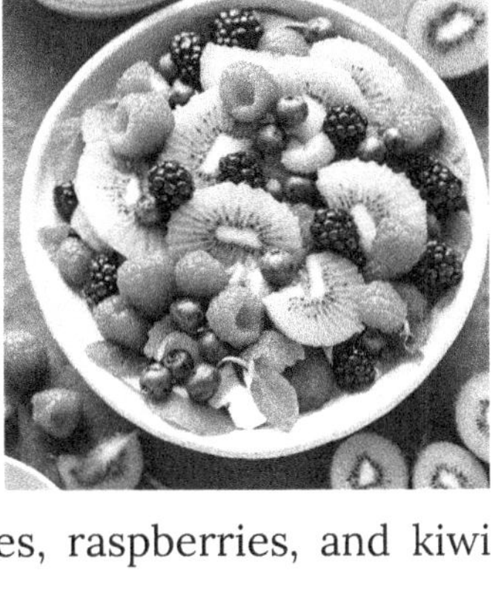

18. Pumpkin Seed Muesli

Ingredients

- 1 cup rolled oats
- 1/2 cup pumpkin seeds
- 1/4 cup chopped almonds
- 1/4 cup chopped dried apricots (unsweetened)
- 1/4 cup raisins (unsweetened)
- 1 tablespoon chia seeds
- 1 teaspoon ground cinnamon
- 1 cup almond milk (unsweetened), for serving

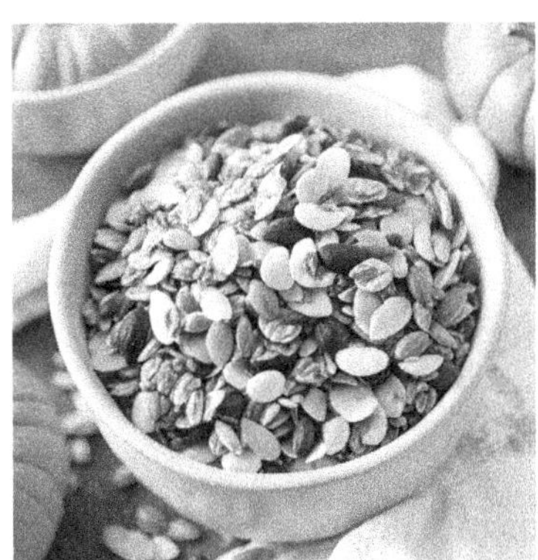

Instructions

1. In a large bowl, combine the rolled oats, pumpkin seeds, chopped almonds, chopped dried apricots, raisins, chia seeds, and ground cinnamon.
2. Mix well to combine.
3. Store the muesli in an airtight container.
4. To serve, place 1/2 cup of the muesli in a bowl and pour 1 cup of almond milk over it.
5. Let it sit for a few minutes to soften, then enjoy.

Nutrition Info per Serving

Calories: 250   Protein: 8g   Fat: 12g   Carbohydrates: 30g Fiber: 6gSugar: 12g

Serves 4

Cooking Time

5 minutes (plus soaking time)

19. Millet Porridge

Ingredients

- 1 cup millet
- 3 cups water
- 1 cup almond milk (unsweetened)
- 1 tablespoon honey
- 1 teaspoon ground cinnamon
- 1/2 teaspoon ground ginger
- 1/4 cup chopped pecans (optional)
- Fresh berries for topping (optional)

Instructions

1. Rinse the millet under cold water.
2. In a medium saucepan, combine the millet and water. Bring to a boil over medium-high heat.
3. Reduce the heat to low, cover, and simmer for about 20 minutes until the millet is tender and the water is absorbed.
4. Stir in the almond milk, honey, ground cinnamon, and ground ginger.
5. Cook for an additional 5 minutes, stirring occasionally, until the porridge is creamy.
6. Serve hot, topped with chopped pecans and fresh berries if desired.

Nutrition Info per Serving

- Calories: 230
- Protein: 6g
- Fat: 6g
- Carbohydrates: 38g
- Fiber: 4g
- Sugar: 9g

Serves

4

Cooking Time

30 minutes

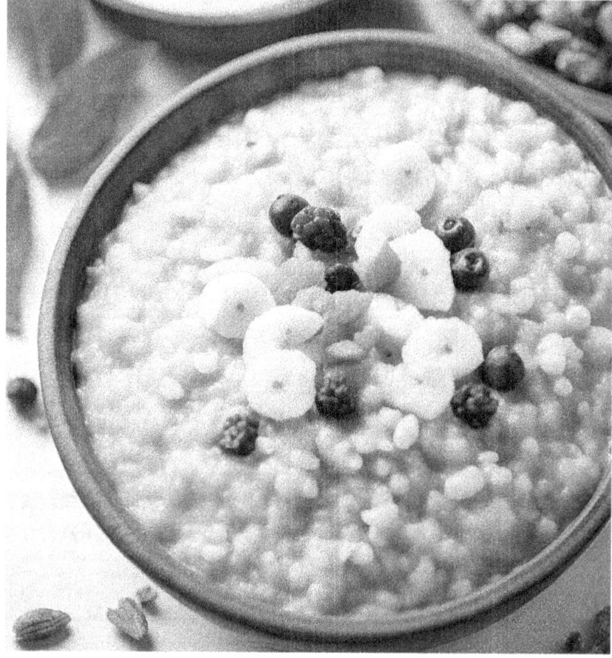

20. Vegan Breakfast Tacos

Ingredients

- 1 tablespoon olive oil
- 1/2 cup diced onion
- 1 red bell pepper, diced
- 1 yellow bell pepper, diced
- 1 can (15 ounces) black beans, drained and rinsed
- 1 teaspoon ground cumin
- 1 teaspoon ground paprika
- 1/2 teaspoon ground turmeric
- 4 small corn tortillas
- 1 avocado, sliced
- 1/4 cup chopped cilantro
- Lime wedges (optional)

Instructions

1. Heat the olive oil in a skillet over medium heat.
2. Add the diced onion and bell peppers, and sauté for about 5 minutes until they are softened.
3. Stir in the black beans, cumin, paprika, and turmeric. Cook for an additional 5 minutes until everything is heated through.
4. Warm the corn tortillas in a dry skillet or microwave.
5. Divide the bean and pepper mixture evenly among the tortillas.
6. Top each taco with sliced avocado and chopped cilantro.
7. Serve with lime wedges if desired.

Nutrition Info per Serving

- Calories: 260
- Protein: 8g
- Fat: 12g
- Carbohydrates: 33g
- Fiber: 10g
- Sugar: 3g

Serves

4

Cooking Time

15 minutes

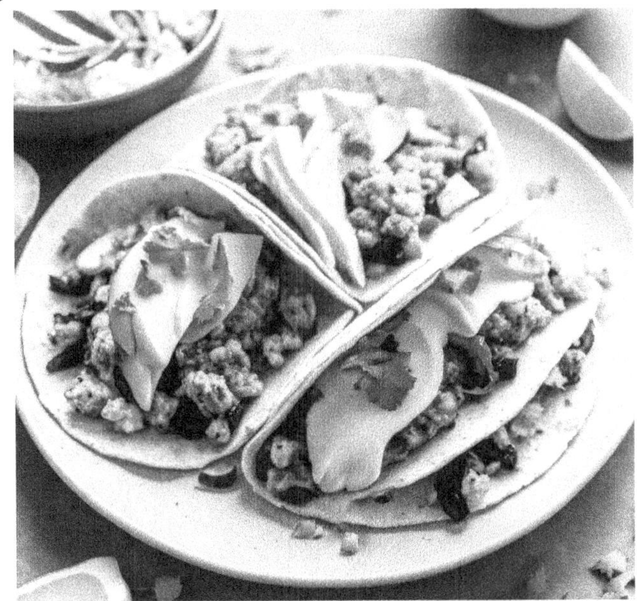

21. Almond Yogurt with Honey and Walnuts

Ingredients

- 2 cups almond yogurt (unsweetened)
- 2 tablespoons honey
- 1/4 cup chopped walnuts
- 1/2 teaspoon ground cinnamon

Instructions

1. Divide the almond yogurt into two bowls.
2. Drizzle each serving with 1 tablespoon of honey.
3. Sprinkle with chopped walnuts and ground cinnamon.
4. Serve immediately.

Nutrition Info per Serving

- Calories: 200 Protein: 5g Fat: 10g   Carbohydrates: 25g   Fiber: 2g Sugar: 18g

Serves 2

Cooking Time

5 minutes

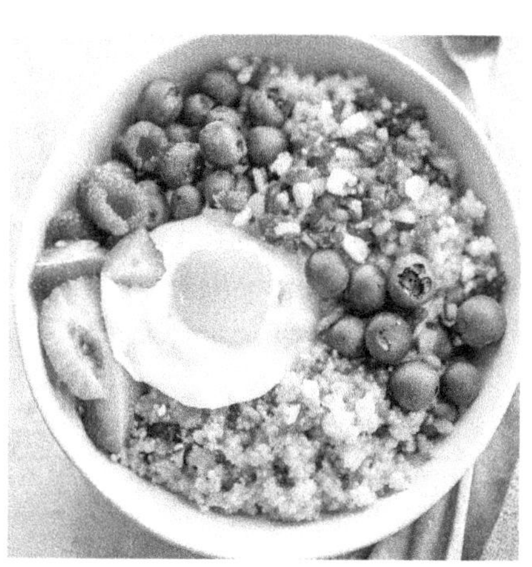

22. Quinoa Breakfast Bowl

Ingredients

- 1 cup quinoa, rinsed
- 2 cups water
- 1 cup almond milk (unsweetened)
- 1 tablespoon maple syrup
- 1 teaspoon ground cinnamon
- 1/4 cup sliced almonds
- 1/4 cup fresh blueberries

Instructions

1. In a medium saucepan, combine the quinoa and water. Bring to a boil over medium-high heat.
2. Reduce heat to low, cover, and simmer for about 15 minutes until the quinoa is tender and the water is absorbed.
3. Stir in the almond milk, maple syrup, and ground cinnamon. Cook for an additional 5 minutes, stirring occasionally.
4. Serve the quinoa in bowls, topped with sliced almonds and fresh blueberries.

Nutrition Info per Serving

- Calories: 280 Protein: 9g Fat: 9g Carbohydrates: 42g Fiber: 5g
- Sugar: 10g

Serves 2

Cooking Time

20 minutes

23. Turmeric Porridge

Ingredients

- 1 cup rolled oats
- 2 cups almond milk (unsweetened)
- 1 teaspoon ground turmeric
- 1/2 teaspoon ground cinnamon
- 1 tablespoon honey
- 1/4 cup raisins

Instructions

1. In a medium saucepan, combine the rolled oats, almond milk, turmeric, and cinnamon. Bring to a boil over medium heat.
2. Reduce heat to low and simmer for about 5-7 minutes, stirring occasionally, until the oats are tender and the porridge has thickened.
3. Stir in the honey and raisins.
4. Serve hot.

Nutrition Info per Serving

- Calories: 220
- Protein: 5g
- Fat: 5g
- Carbohydrates: 40g
- Fiber: 6g
- Sugar: 15g

Serves 2
Cooking Time
10 minutes

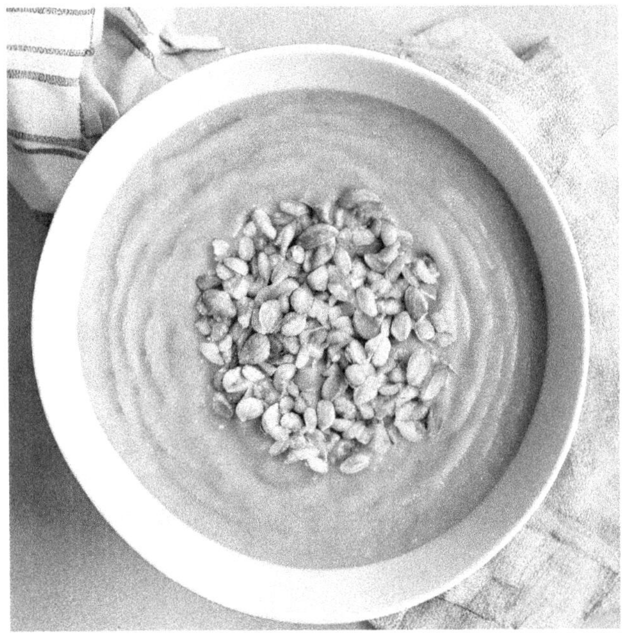

24. Buckwheat Pancakes

Ingredients

- 1 cup buckwheat flour
- 1 teaspoon baking powder
- 1 teaspoon ground cinnamon
- 1 cup almond milk (unsweetened)
- 1 tablespoon maple syrup
- 1 teaspoon vanilla extract
- 1 tablespoon coconut oil, melted

Instructions

1. In a large bowl, mix the buckwheat flour, baking powder, and ground cinnamon.
2. In another bowl, whisk together the almond milk, maple syrup, vanilla extract, and melted coconut oil.
3. Pour the wet ingredients into the dry ingredients and mix until just combined.
4. Heat a non-stick skillet over medium heat and lightly grease with a bit of coconut oil.
5. Pour 1/4 cup of batter onto the skillet and cook for about 2-3 minutes on each side, until bubbles form on the surface and the edges look set.
6. Repeat with the remaining batter.
7. Serve warm with additional maple syrup if desired.

Nutrition Info per Serving

- Calories: 200
- Protein: 5g
- Fat: 7g
- Carbohydrates: 31g
- Fiber: 4g
- Sugar: 6g

Serves

4

Cooking Time

20 minutes

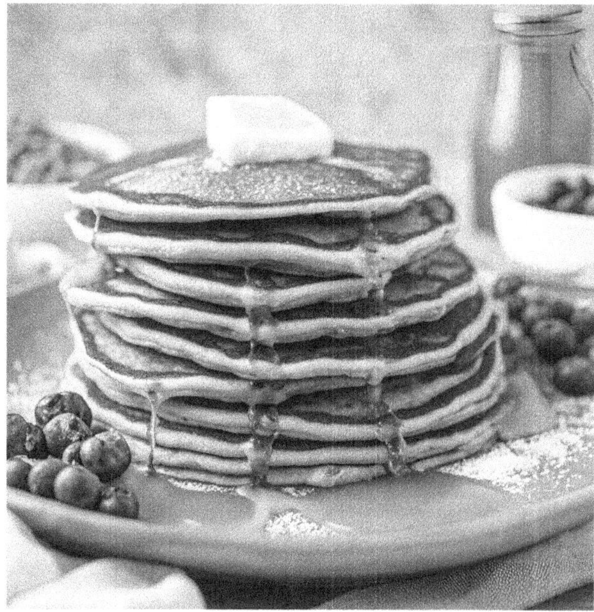

25. Oatmeal with Berries

Ingredients

- 1 cup rolled oats
- 2 cups water
- 1 cup almond milk (unsweetened)
- 1 tablespoon honey
- 1 teaspoon ground cinnamon
- 1 cup mixed berries (blueberries, strawberries, raspberries)
- 1 tablespoon chia seeds

Instructions

1. In a medium saucepan, combine the rolled oats and water. Bring to a boil over medium heat.
2. Reduce heat to low and simmer for about 5 minutes, stirring occasionally, until the oats are tender and the water is mostly absorbed.
3. Stir in the almond milk, honey, and ground cinnamon. Cook for an additional 2 minutes.
4. Remove from heat and stir in the chia seeds.
5. Serve topped with mixed berries.

Nutrition Info per Serving

- Calories: 240
- Protein: 6g
- Fat: 6g
- Carbohydrates: 40g
- Fiber: 8g
- Sugar: 14g

Serves

2

Cooking Time

10 minutes

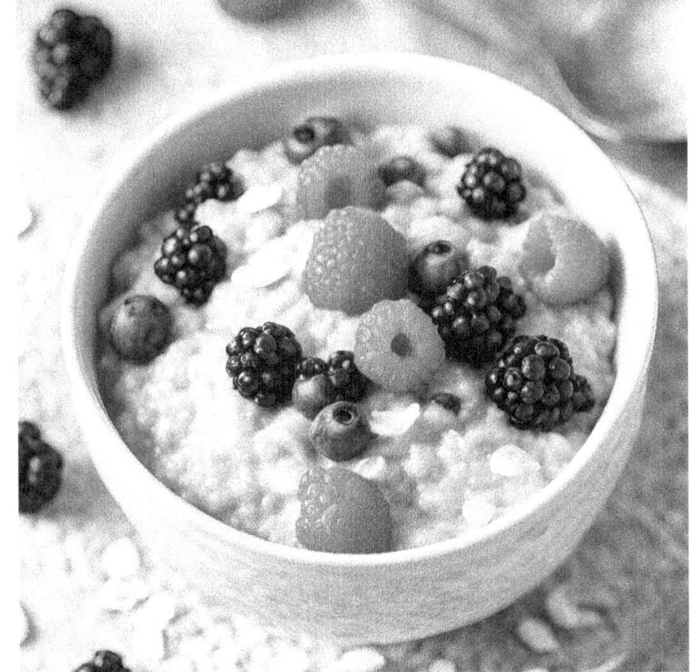

Soup & Stew Recipes

1. Watercress Soup

Ingredients

- 1 tablespoon olive oil
- 1 onion, finely chopped
- 2 cloves garlic, minced
- 4 cups vegetable broth
- 2 large potatoes, peeled and diced
- 4 cups fresh watercress, washed and chopped
- 1 cup unsweetened almond milk
- 1 teaspoon ground nutmeg

Instructions

1. Heat the olive oil in a large pot over medium heat.
2. Add the chopped onion and garlic, and sauté for about 5 minutes until softened.
3. Add the vegetable broth and diced potatoes. Bring to a boil, then reduce heat and simmer for about 15 minutes until the potatoes are tender.
4. Add the chopped watercress and cook for an additional 5 minutes until wilted.
5. Remove from heat and blend the soup until smooth using an immersion blender or in batches in a regular blender.
6. Return the soup to the pot, stir in the almond milk and ground nutmeg, and heat through.
7. Serve hot.

Nutrition Info per Serving

- Calories: 120
- Protein: 3g
- Fat: 4g
- Carbohydrates: 20g
- Fiber: 3g
- Sugar: 3g

Serves

4

Cooking Time

30 minutes

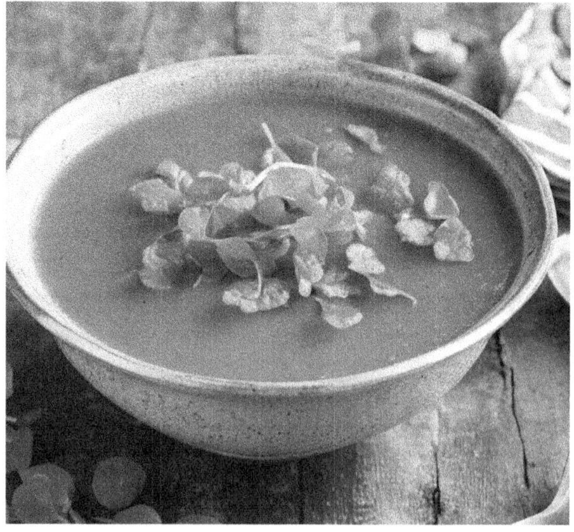

2. Cream of Mushroom Soup

Ingredients

- 2 tablespoons olive oil
- 1 onion, finely chopped
- 3 cloves garlic, minced
- 16 ounces mushrooms, sliced
- 4 cups vegetable broth
- 1 cup unsweetened almond milk
- 2 tablespoons gluten-free flour (such as rice flour)
- 1 teaspoon dried thyme

Instructions

1. Heat the olive oil in a large pot over medium heat.
2. Add the onion and garlic, and sauté for about 5 minutes until softened.
3. Add the sliced mushrooms and cook for about 10 minutes until the mushrooms are browned and their liquid is released.
4. Stir in the gluten-free flour and cook for 2 minutes.
5. Add the vegetable broth and dried thyme. Bring to a boil, then reduce heat and simmer for about 10 minutes.
6. Blend the soup until smooth using an immersion blender or in batches in a regular blender.
7. Return the soup to the pot, stir in the almond milk, and heat through.
8. Serve hot.

Nutrition Info per Serving

- Calories: 150
- Protein: 5g
- Fat: 9g
- Carbohydrates: 15g
- Fiber: 3g
- Sugar: 4g

Serves

4

Cooking Time

30 minutes

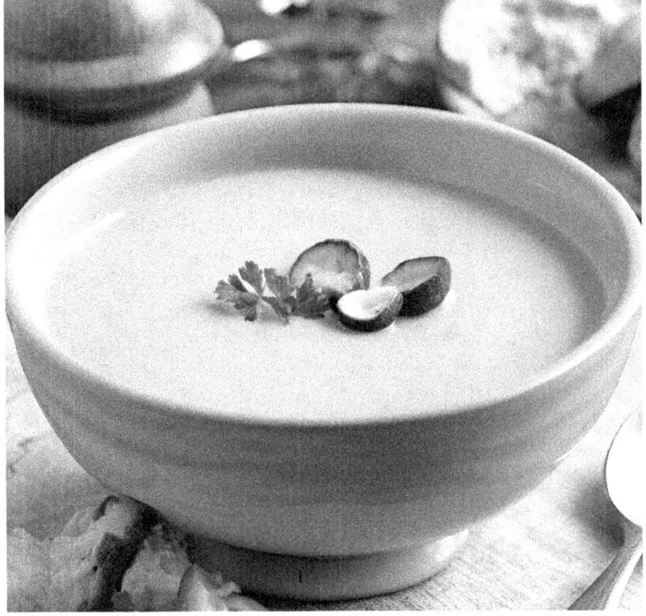

3. Japanese Clear Soup
Ingredients
- 4 cups vegetable broth
- 1 carrot, thinly sliced
- 1 celery stalk, thinly sliced
- 4 mushrooms, thinly sliced
- 2 green onions, thinly sliced
- 1 teaspoon grated ginger
- 1 tablespoon tamari (gluten-free soy sauce)

Instructions
1. In a large pot, bring the vegetable broth to a boil.
2. Add the carrot, celery, mushrooms, green onions, and grated ginger.
3. Reduce heat and simmer for about 10 minutes until the vegetables are tender.
4. Stir in the tamari and cook for an additional 2 minutes.
5. Serve hot.

Nutrition Info per Serving
- Calories: 50
- Protein: 2g
- Fat: 0g
- Carbohydrates: 10g
- Fiber: 2g
- Sugar: 3g

Serves
4

Cooking Time
15 minutes

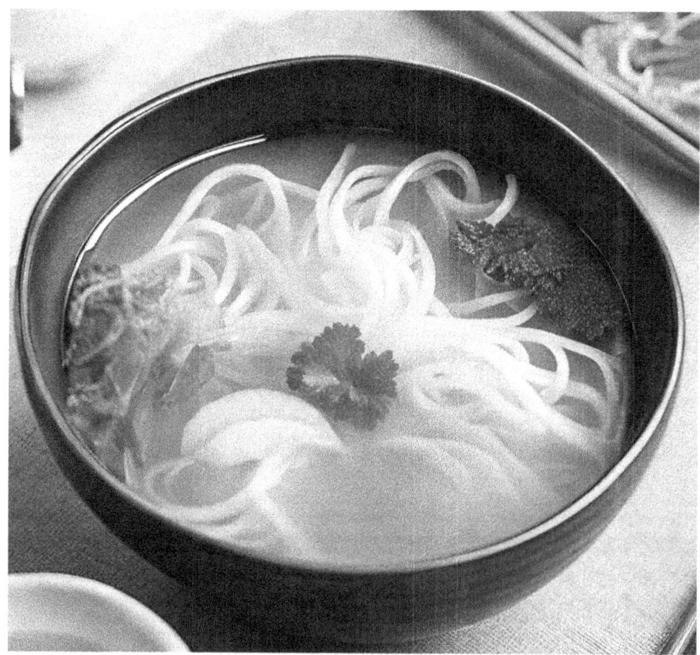

4. Celery Root and Apple Soup
Ingredients
- 2 tablespoons olive oil
- 1 onion, finely chopped
- 2 cloves garlic, minced
- 1 large celery root (celeriac), peeled and diced
- 2 apples, peeled, cored, and diced
- 4 cups vegetable broth
- 1 cup unsweetened almond milk
- 1 teaspoon ground nutmeg

Instructions
1. Heat the olive oil in a large pot over medium heat.
2. Add the onion and garlic, and sauté for about 5 minutes until softened.
3. Add the diced celery root and apples. Cook for about 10 minutes, stirring occasionally.
4. Add the vegetable broth and bring to a boil. Reduce heat and simmer for about 20 minutes until the celery root is tender.
5. Blend the soup until smooth using an immersion blender or in batches in a regular blender.
6. Return the soup to the pot, stir in the almond milk and ground nutmeg, and heat through.
7. Serve hot.

Nutrition Info per Serving
- Calories: 140
- Protein: 2g
- Fat: 7g
- Carbohydrates: 20g
- Fiber: 4g
- Sugar: 10g

Serves
4

Cooking Time
35 minutes

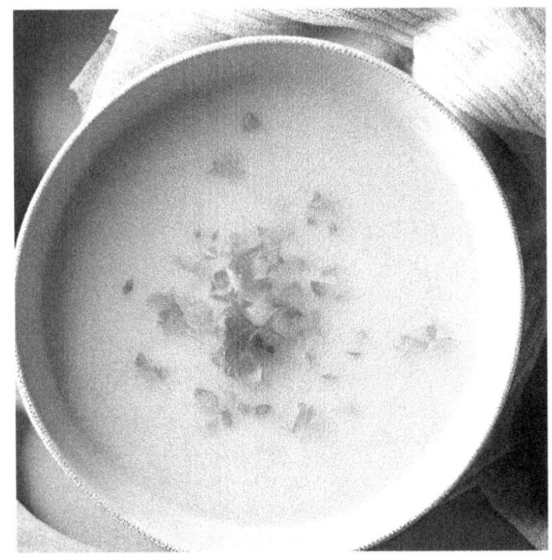

5. Caribbean Chickpea and Potato Curry

Ingredients

- 1 tablespoon coconut oil
- 1 onion, finely chopped
- 3 cloves garlic, minced
- 1-inch piece of ginger, grated
- 1 tablespoon curry powder
- 1 teaspoon ground turmeric
- 1 teaspoon ground cumin
- 1 can (15 ounces) chickpeas, drained and rinsed
- 2 large potatoes, peeled and diced
- 1 can (14 ounces) coconut milk
- 1 cup vegetable broth
- 1 cup spinach, chopped
- 1 tablespoon lime juice

Instructions

1. Heat the coconut oil in a large pot over medium heat.
2. Add the onion, garlic, and grated ginger, and sauté for about 5 minutes until softened.
3. Stir in the curry powder, turmeric, and cumin, and cook for an additional 2 minutes.
4. Add the chickpeas, potatoes, coconut milk, and vegetable broth. Bring to a boil, then reduce heat and simmer for about 20 minutes until the potatoes are tender.
5. Stir in the chopped spinach and cook for an additional 5 minutes until wilted.
6. Remove from heat and stir in the lime juice.
7. Serve hot.

Nutrition Info per Serving

- Calories: 320
- Protein: 8g
- Fat: 16g
- Carbohydrates: 40g
- Fiber: 8g
- Sugar: 4g

Serves

4

Cooking Time

35 minutes

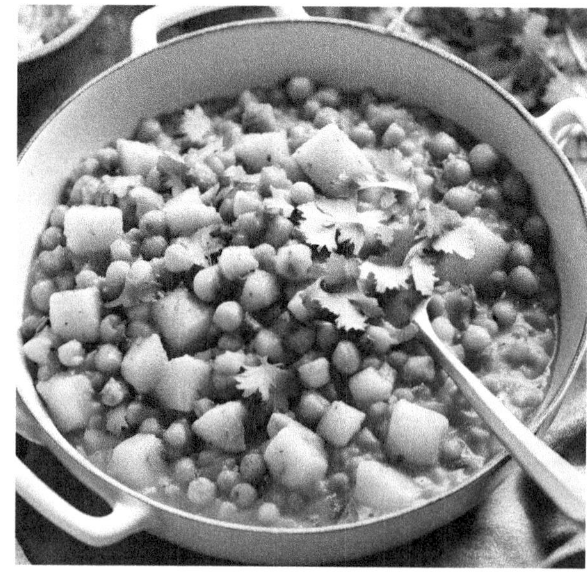

6. Squash and Apple Stew

Ingredients

- 2 tablespoons olive oil
- 1 large onion, finely chopped
- 2 cloves garlic, minced
- 1 butternut squash, peeled, seeded, and cubed
- 2 apples, peeled, cored, and cubed
- 4 cups vegetable broth
- 1 teaspoon ground cinnamon
- 1/2 teaspoon ground nutmeg
- 1/2 teaspoon ground ginger
- 1/4 cup chopped fresh parsley

Instructions

1. Heat the olive oil in a large pot over medium heat.
2. Add the onion and garlic, and sauté for about 5 minutes until softened.
3. Add the cubed butternut squash and apples. Cook for about 10 minutes, stirring occasionally.
4. Stir in the vegetable broth, cinnamon, nutmeg, and ground ginger. Bring to a boil, then reduce heat and simmer for about 20 minutes until the squash and apples are tender.
5. Use an immersion blender to blend the stew to your desired consistency, or blend in batches in a regular blender.
6. Stir in the chopped parsley and cook for another 2 minutes.
7. Serve hot.

Nutrition Info per Serving

- Calories: 180
- Protein: 2g
- Fat: 7g
- Carbohydrates: 31g
- Fiber: 6g
- Sugar: 10g

Serves

4

Cooking Time

35 minutes

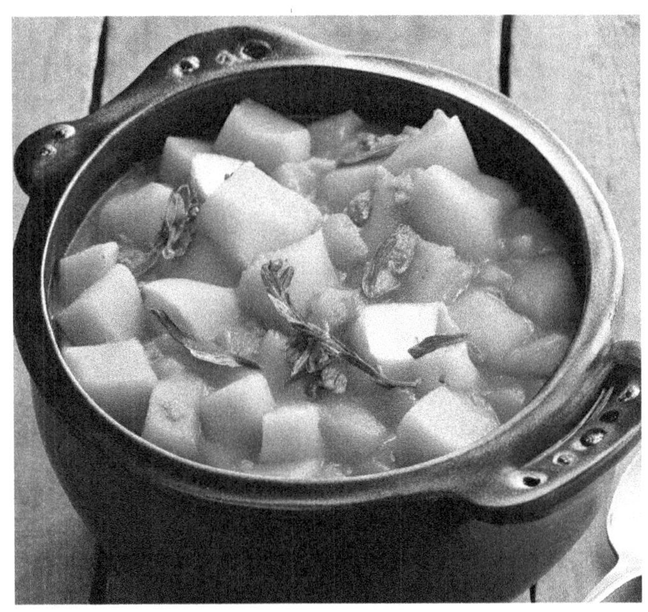

7. Asparagus and Lemon Soup

Ingredients

- 2 tablespoons olive oil
- 1 onion, finely chopped
- 2 cloves garlic, minced
- 1 pound asparagus, trimmed and chopped
- 4 cups vegetable broth
- 1 cup unsweetened almond milk
- 1 teaspoon grated lemon zest
- 2 tablespoons lemon juice
- 1/4 cup chopped fresh dill

Instructions

1. Heat the olive oil in a large pot over medium heat.
2. Add the onion and garlic, and sauté for about 5 minutes until softened.
3. Add the chopped asparagus and cook for about 5 minutes.
4. Stir in the vegetable broth and bring to a boil. Reduce heat and simmer for about 10 minutes until the asparagus is tender.
5. Use an immersion blender to blend the soup until smooth, or blend in batches in a regular blender.
6. Stir in the almond milk, lemon zest, and lemon juice. Cook for another 2 minutes until heated through.
7. Serve hot, garnished with fresh dill.

Nutrition Info per Serving

- Calories: 120
- Protein: 4g
- Fat: 7g
- Carbohydrates: 13g
- Fiber: 4g
- Sugar: 5g

Serves

4

Cooking Time

25 minutes

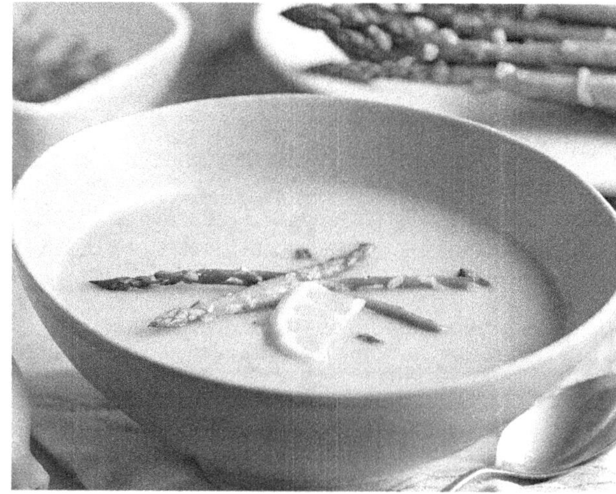

8. Kale and Sausage Stew

Ingredients

- 1 tablespoon olive oil
- 1 pound turkey or chicken sausage, sliced
- 1 onion, finely chopped
- 2 cloves garlic, minced
- 1 bunch kale, stems removed and leaves chopped
- 4 cups vegetable broth
- 2 large potatoes, peeled and diced
- 1 teaspoon ground paprika
- 1/2 teaspoon ground cumin
- 1/4 cup chopped fresh parsley

Instructions

1. Heat the olive oil in a large pot over medium heat.
2. Add the sausage slices and cook for about 5 minutes until browned.
3. Add the onion and garlic, and sauté for another 5 minutes until softened.
4. Stir in the chopped kale, vegetable broth, and diced potatoes. Add the paprika and cumin.
5. Bring to a boil, then reduce heat and simmer for about 20 minutes until the potatoes are tender.
6. Stir in the chopped parsley and cook for another 2 minutes.
7. Serve hot.

Nutrition Info per Serving

- Calories: 280
- Protein: 20g
- Fat: 12g
- Carbohydrates: 25g
- Fiber: 5g
- Sugar: 4g

Serves

4

Cooking Time

35 minutes

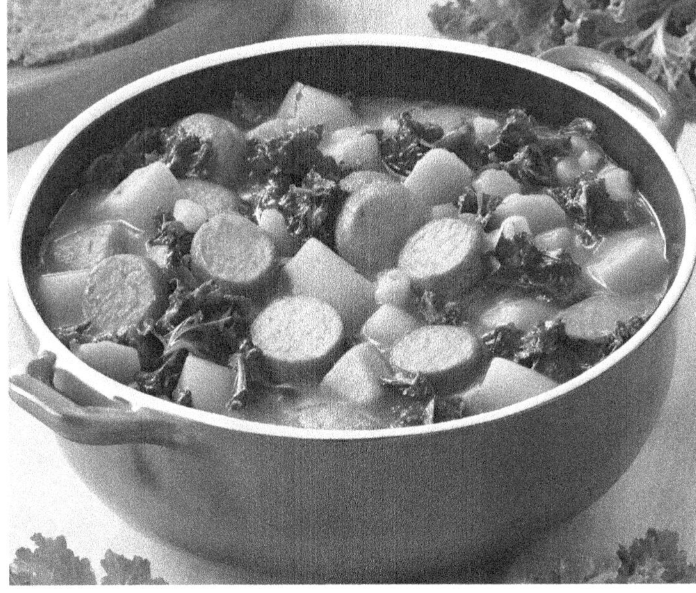

9. Vegan Mushroom Stroganoff Soup

Ingredients

- 2 tablespoons olive oil
- 1 onion, finely chopped
- 3 cloves garlic, minced
- 16 ounces mushrooms, sliced
- 4 cups vegetable broth
- 1 cup unsweetened almond milk
- 2 tablespoons gluten-free flour (such as rice flour)
- 1 teaspoon dried thyme
- 1 tablespoon nutritional yeast
- 1/4 cup chopped fresh parsley

Instructions

1. Heat the olive oil in a large pot over medium heat.
2. Add the onion and garlic, and sauté for about 5 minutes until softened.
3. Add the sliced mushrooms and cook for about 10 minutes until the mushrooms are browned and their liquid is released.
4. Stir in the gluten-free flour and cook for 2 minutes.
5. Add the vegetable broth, dried thyme, and nutritional yeast. Bring to a boil, then reduce heat and simmer for about 10 minutes.
6. Blend the soup until smooth using an immersion blender or in batches in a regular blender.
7. Return the soup to the pot, stir in the almond milk, and heat through.
8. Serve hot, garnished with fresh parsley.

Nutrition Info per Serving

- Calories: 180
- Protein: 6g
- Fat: 10g
- Carbohydrates: 18g
- Fiber: 4g
- Sugar: 3g

Serves

4

Cooking Time

30 minutes

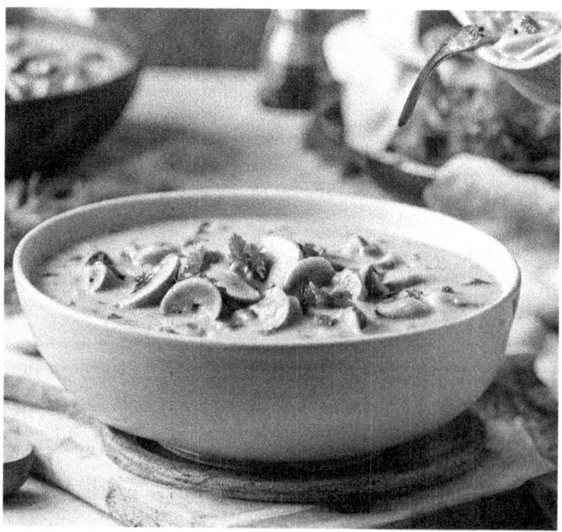

10. Fish Stew with Tomatoes

Ingredients

- 1 tablespoon olive oil
- 1 onion, finely chopped
- 2 cloves garlic, minced
- 1 red bell pepper, chopped
- 1 can (14 ounces) diced tomatoes
- 4 cups vegetable broth
- 1 pound white fish fillets (such as cod or tilapia), cut into chunks
- 1 teaspoon dried oregano
- 1 teaspoon smoked paprika
- 1/4 cup chopped fresh cilantro

Instructions

1. Heat the olive oil in a large pot over medium heat.
2. Add the onion, garlic, and red bell pepper, and sauté for about 5 minutes until softened.
3. Stir in the diced tomatoes, vegetable broth, dried oregano, and smoked paprika. Bring to a boil, then reduce heat and simmer for about 10 minutes.
4. Add the fish chunks and cook for about 5 minutes until the fish is cooked through and flakes easily with a fork.
5. Stir in the chopped cilantro and cook for another 2 minutes.
6. Serve hot.

Nutrition Info per Serving

- Calories: 220
- Protein: 24g
- Fat: 8g
- Carbohydrates: 14g
- Fiber: 3g
- Sugar: 6g

Serves

4

Cooking Time

25 minutes

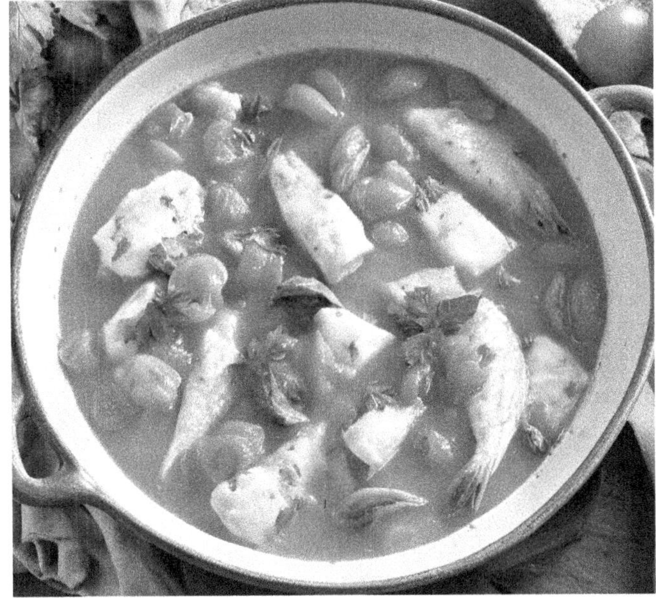

11. Apple and Parsnip Soup

Ingredients

- 2 tablespoons olive oil
- 1 large onion, finely chopped
- 2 cloves garlic, minced
- 4 parsnips, peeled and chopped
- 2 apples, peeled, cored, and chopped
- 4 cups vegetable broth
- 1 teaspoon ground cumin
- 1/2 teaspoon ground cinnamon
- 1/4 teaspoon ground nutmeg
- 1 cup unsweetened almond milk

Instructions

1. Heat the olive oil in a large pot over medium heat.
2. Add the onion and garlic, and sauté for about 5 minutes until softened.
3. Add the chopped parsnips and apples. Cook for about 10 minutes, stirring occasionally.
4. Stir in the vegetable broth, ground cumin, cinnamon, and nutmeg. Bring to a boil, then reduce heat and simmer for about 20 minutes until the parsnips are tender.
5. Use an immersion blender to blend the soup until smooth, or blend in batches in a regular blender.
6. Stir in the almond milk and heat through.
7. Serve hot.

Nutrition Info per Serving

- Calories: 190
- Protein: 2g
- Fat: 8g
- Carbohydrates: 28g
- Fiber: 6g
- Sugar: 12g

Serves

4

Cooking Time

35 minutes

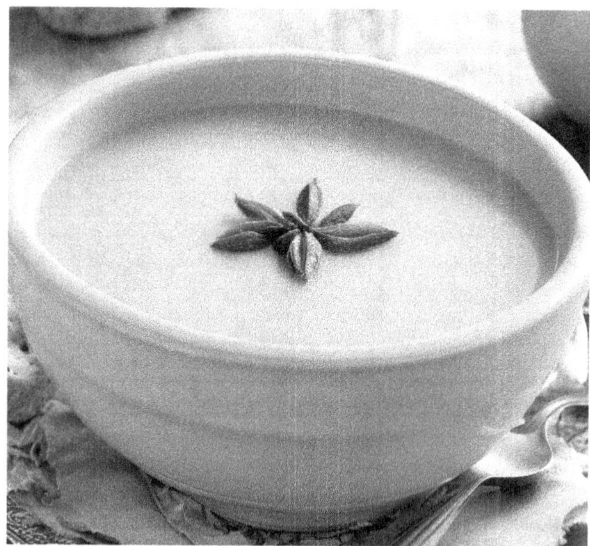

12. Roasted Red Pepper Soup

Ingredients

- 6 red bell peppers
- 2 tablespoons olive oil
- 1 large onion, finely chopped
- 3 cloves garlic, minced
- 4 cups vegetable broth
- 1 teaspoon smoked paprika
- 1 cup unsweetened almond milk

Instructions

1. Preheat the oven to 400°F (200°C). Place the red bell peppers on a baking sheet and roast for 25-30 minutes, turning occasionally, until the skins are blackened and blistered.
2. Remove the peppers from the oven and place them in a covered bowl to steam for about 10 minutes. Peel off the skins, remove the seeds, and chop the peppers.
3. In a large pot, heat the olive oil over medium heat. Add the onion and garlic, and sauté for about 5 minutes until softened.
4. Add the roasted red peppers, vegetable broth, and smoked paprika. Bring to a boil, then reduce heat and simmer for about 10 minutes.
5. Use an immersion blender to blend the soup until smooth, or blend in batches in a regular blender.
6. Stir in the almond milk and heat through.
7. Serve hot.

Nutrition Info per Serving

- Calories: 160
- Protein: 3g
- Fat: 8g
- Carbohydrates: 20g
- Fiber: 4g
- Sugar: 10g

Serves

4

Cooking Time

45 minutes

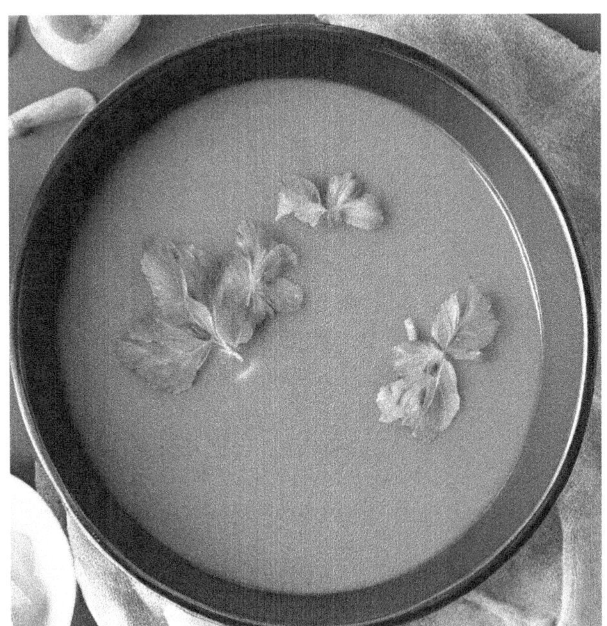

13. Thai Coconut Shrimp Soup

Ingredients

- 1 tablespoon coconut oil
- 1 onion, finely chopped
- 2 cloves garlic, minced
- 1 tablespoon grated ginger
- 1 tablespoon red curry paste
- 4 cups vegetable broth
- 1 can (14 ounces) coconut milk
- 1 pound shrimp, peeled and deveined
- 1 red bell pepper, thinly sliced
- 2 cups baby spinach
- 2 tablespoons lime juice
- 1/4 cup chopped fresh cilantro

Instructions

1. Heat the coconut oil in a large pot over medium heat.
2. Add the onion, garlic, and grated ginger, and sauté for about 5 minutes until softened.
3. Stir in the red curry paste and cook for 2 minutes.
4. Add the vegetable broth and coconut milk. Bring to a boil, then reduce heat and simmer for about 10 minutes.
5. Add the shrimp and red bell pepper, and cook for about 5 minutes until the shrimp is cooked through.
6. Stir in the baby spinach and cook until wilted.
7. Remove from heat and stir in the lime juice.
8. Serve hot, garnished with fresh cilantro.

Nutrition Info per Serving

- Calories: 300
- Protein: 20g
- Fat: 20g
- Carbohydrates: 12g
- Fiber: 3g
- Sugar: 5g

Serves

4

Cooking Time

30 minutes

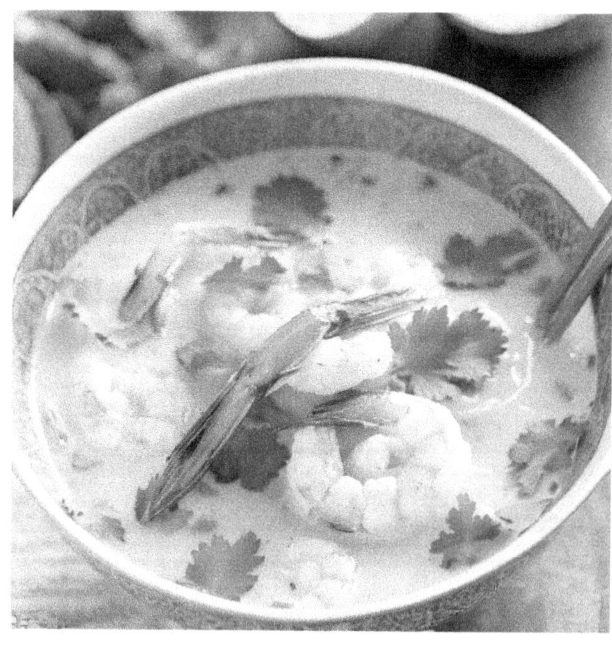

14. Cauliflower and Hemp Seed Soup

Ingredients

- 2 tablespoons olive oil
- 1 large onion, finely chopped
- 2 cloves garlic, minced
- 1 large cauliflower, chopped
- 4 cups vegetable broth
- 1 cup unsweetened almond milk
- 1/4 cup hemp seeds
- 1 teaspoon ground turmeric
- 1/4 cup chopped fresh parsley

Instructions

1. Heat the olive oil in a large pot over medium heat.
2. Add the onion and garlic, and sauté for about 5 minutes until softened.
3. Add the chopped cauliflower, vegetable broth, and ground turmeric. Bring to a boil, then reduce heat and simmer for about 20 minutes until the cauliflower is tender.
4. Use an immersion blender to blend the soup until smooth, or blend in batches in a regular blender.
5. Stir in the almond milk and hemp seeds, and heat through.
6. Serve hot, garnished with fresh parsley.

Nutrition Info per Serving

- Calories: 200
- Protein: 7g
- Fat: 12g
- Carbohydrates: 18g
- Fiber: 6g
- Sugar: 5g

Serves

4

Cooking Time

30 minutes

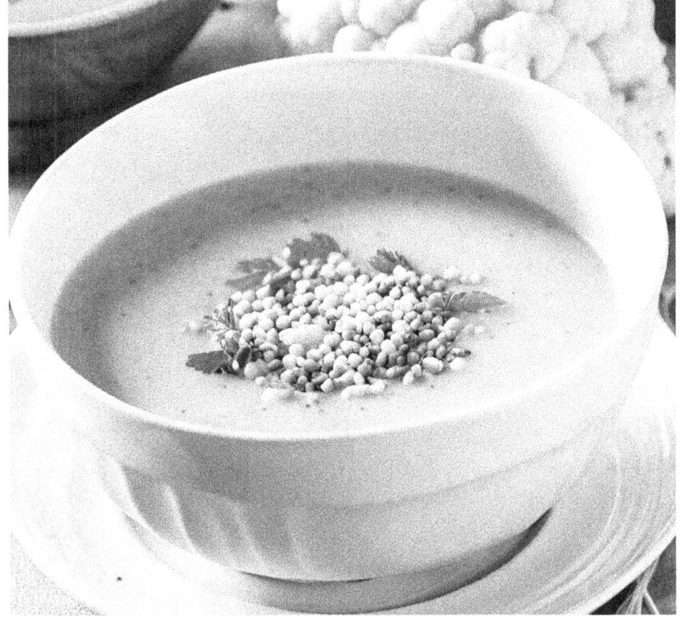

15. Salmon and Sweet Potato Stew
Ingredients

- 1 tablespoon olive oil
- 1 large onion, finely chopped
- 2 cloves garlic, minced
- 1 teaspoon ground paprika
- 1 teaspoon ground cumin
- 4 cups vegetable broth
- 2 large sweet potatoes, peeled and diced
- 1 pound salmon fillets, cut into chunks
- 1 can (14 ounces) diced tomatoes
- 2 cups kale, chopped
- 2 tablespoons lemon juice
- 1/4 cup chopped fresh dill

Instructions

1. Heat the olive oil in a large pot over medium heat.
2. Add the onion and garlic, and sauté for about 5 minutes until softened.
3. Stir in the ground paprika and cumin, and cook for 2 minutes.
4. Add the vegetable broth and diced sweet potatoes. Bring to a boil, then reduce heat and simmer for about 15 minutes until the sweet potatoes are tender.
5. Add the salmon chunks, diced tomatoes, and chopped kale. Cook for about 5-7 minutes until the salmon is cooked through and the kale is wilted.
6. Remove from heat and stir in the lemon juice.
7. Serve hot, garnished with fresh dill.

Nutrition Info per Serving

- Calories: 320
- Protein: 25g
- Fat: 12g
- Carbohydrates: 28g
- Fiber: 6g
- Sugar: 8g

Serves
4
Cooking Time
35 minutes

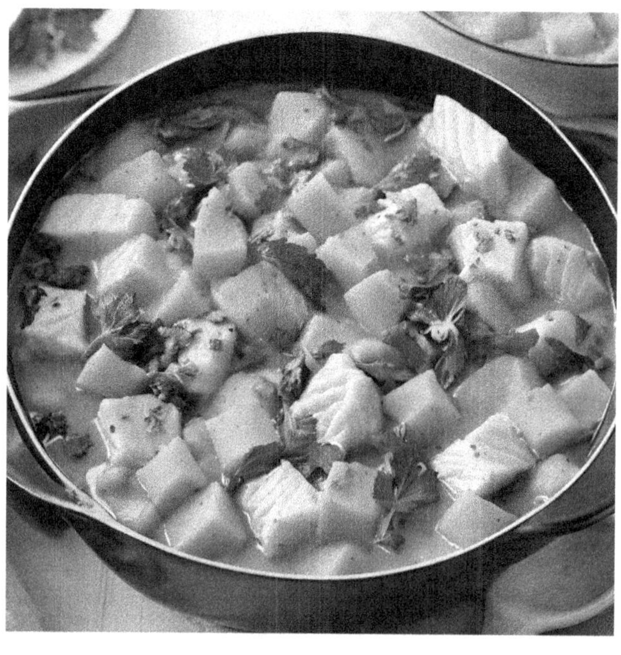

Fish & Seafood Recipes

1. Grilled Salmon with Dill Sauce
Ingredients
- 4 salmon fillets (about 6 ounces each)
- 2 tablespoons olive oil
- 1 tablespoon lemon juice
- 1 teaspoon dried dill weed
- 1 cup plain Greek yogurt
- 1 tablespoon fresh dill, chopped
- 1 tablespoon lemon juice
- 1 clove garlic, minced

Instructions
1. Preheat the grill to medium-high heat.
2. In a small bowl, mix the olive oil, lemon juice, and dried dill weed.
3. Brush the salmon fillets with the olive oil mixture.
4. Grill the salmon for about 4-5 minutes on each side, until the fish flakes easily with a fork.
5. While the salmon is grilling, prepare the dill sauce. In a small bowl, mix the Greek yogurt, fresh dill, lemon juice, and minced garlic.
6. Serve the grilled salmon hot, topped with the dill sauce.

Nutrition Info per Serving
- Calories: 320
- Protein: 34g
- Fat: 18g
- Carbohydrates: 4g
- Fiber: 0g
- Sugar: 2g

Serves
4

Cooking Time
20 minutes

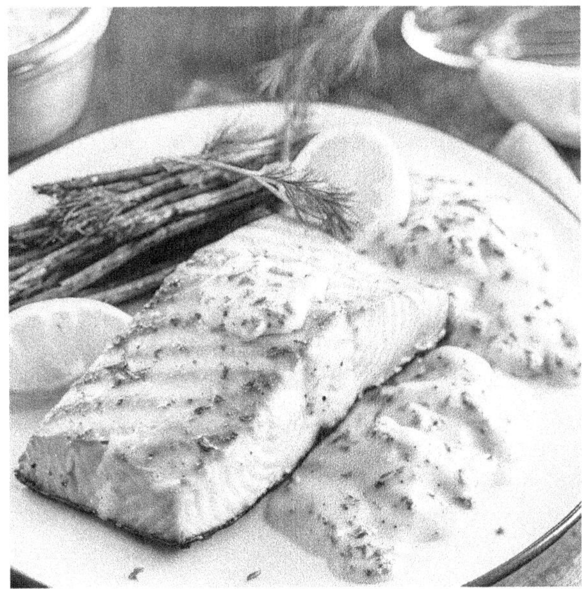

2. Herb-Crusted Cod

Ingredients

- 4 cod fillets (about 6 ounces each)
- 1/2 cup almond flour
- 1/4 cup chopped fresh parsley
- 1 tablespoon chopped fresh thyme
- 1 tablespoon chopped fresh rosemary
- 2 cloves garlic, minced
- 2 tablespoons olive oil
- 1 tablespoon lemon juice

Instructions

1. Preheat the oven to 375°F (190°C). Line a baking sheet with parchment paper.
2. In a bowl, combine the almond flour, chopped parsley, thyme, rosemary, and minced garlic.
3. Brush the cod fillets with olive oil and lemon juice.
4. Press the herb mixture onto the cod fillets, coating them evenly.
5. Place the fillets on the prepared baking sheet and bake for about 15-20 minutes, until the fish is cooked through and flakes easily with a fork.
6. Serve hot.

Nutrition Info per Serving

- Calories: 290
- Protein: 34g
- Fat: 14g
- Carbohydrates: 6g
- Fiber: 2g
- Sugar: 0g

Serves

4

Cooking Time

25 minutes

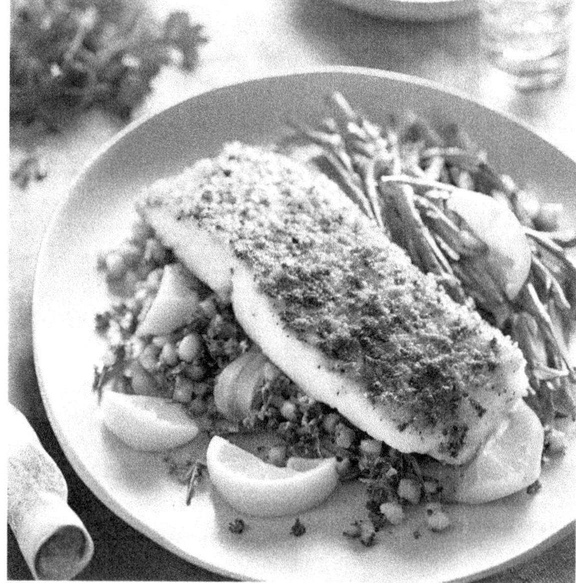

3. Shrimp Stir-Fry

Ingredients

- 1 tablespoon coconut oil
- 1 pound large shrimp, peeled and deveined
- 1 red bell pepper, sliced
- 1 yellow bell pepper, sliced
- 1 zucchini, sliced
- 1 cup snap peas
- 2 cloves garlic, minced
- 1 tablespoon grated ginger
- 2 tablespoons tamari (gluten-free soy sauce)
- 1 tablespoon sesame oil
- 1 tablespoon sesame seeds

Instructions

1. Heat the coconut oil in a large skillet or wok over medium-high heat.
2. Add the shrimp and cook for about 2-3 minutes until pink and opaque. Remove shrimp from the skillet and set aside.
3. In the same skillet, add the red and yellow bell peppers, zucchini, and snap peas. Cook for about 5 minutes until tender-crisp.
4. Add the minced garlic and grated ginger, and cook for another 2 minutes.
5. Return the shrimp to the skillet and stir in the tamari and sesame oil. Cook for another 2 minutes until everything is heated through.
6. Sprinkle with sesame seeds and serve hot.

Nutrition Info per Serving

- Calories: 240
- Protein: 28g
- Fat: 10g
- Carbohydrates: 10g
- Fiber: 3g
- Sugar: 4g

Serves

4

Cooking Time

15 minutes

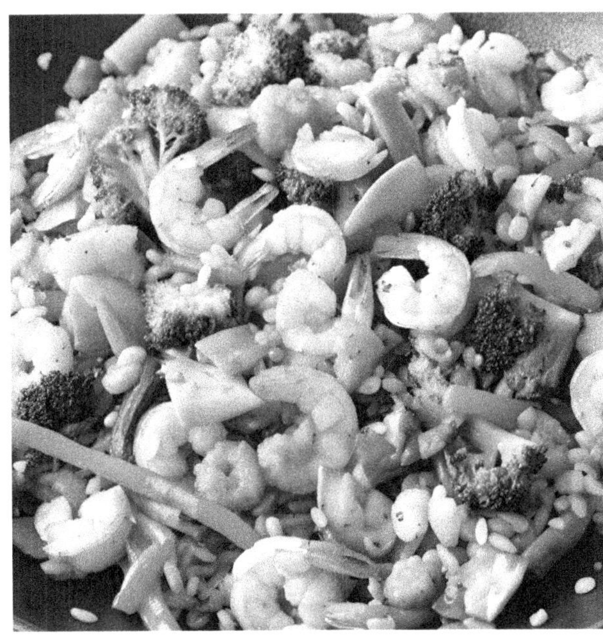

4. Tuna and Avocado Salad
Ingredients

- 2 cans (5 ounces each) tuna packed in water, drained
- 1 avocado, diced
- 1/4 cup red onion, finely chopped
- 1/4 cup fresh cilantro, chopped
- 2 tablespoons lime juice
- 1 tablespoon olive oil
- 1 teaspoon ground cumin

Instructions

1. In a large bowl, combine the drained tuna, diced avocado, red onion, and chopped cilantro.
2. In a small bowl, whisk together the lime juice, olive oil, and ground cumin.
3. Pour the dressing over the tuna mixture and gently toss to combine.
4. Serve immediately.

Nutrition Info per Serving

- Calories: 210
- Protein: 20g
- Fat: 14g
- Carbohydrates: 6g
- Fiber: 4g
- Sugar: 1g

Serves
2
Cooking Time
10 minutes

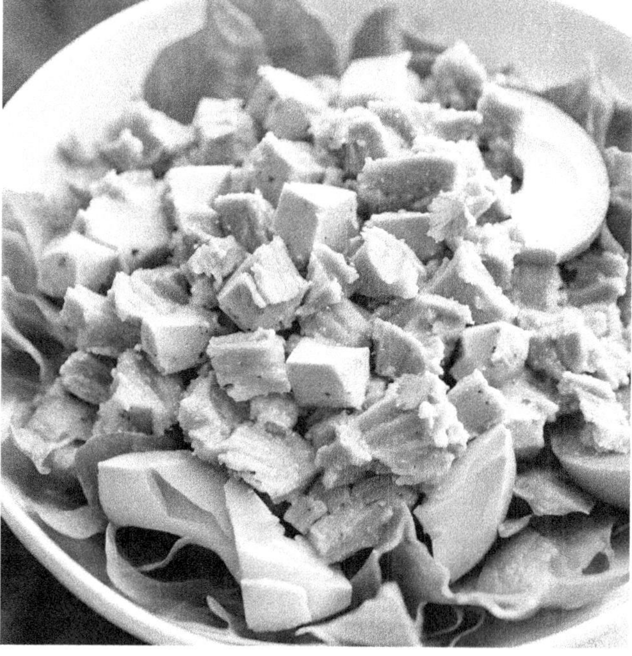

5. Lemon Garlic Shrimp Pasta

Ingredients

- 8 ounces gluten-free pasta
- 2 tablespoons olive oil
- 1 pound large shrimp, peeled and deveined
- 4 cloves garlic, minced
- 1/4 cup lemon juice
- 1 teaspoon lemon zest
- 1/4 cup fresh parsley, chopped
- 1/4 teaspoon red pepper flakes (optional)
- 1 cup cherry tomatoes, halved

Instructions

1. Cook the gluten-free pasta according to package instructions. Drain and set aside.
2. In a large skillet, heat the olive oil over medium heat.
3. Add the shrimp and cook for about 2-3 minutes until they turn pink and are cooked through. Remove the shrimp from the skillet and set aside.
4. In the same skillet, add the minced garlic and cook for about 1 minute until fragrant.
5. Stir in the lemon juice, lemon zest, and cherry tomatoes. Cook for another 2 minutes.
6. Return the shrimp to the skillet and add the cooked pasta. Toss to combine.
7. Sprinkle with fresh parsley and red pepper flakes (if using).
8. Serve hot.

Nutrition Info per Serving

- Calories: 350
- Protein: 28g
- Fat: 10g
- Carbohydrates: 40g
- Fiber: 4g
- Sugar: 3g

Serves

4

Cooking Time

20 minutes

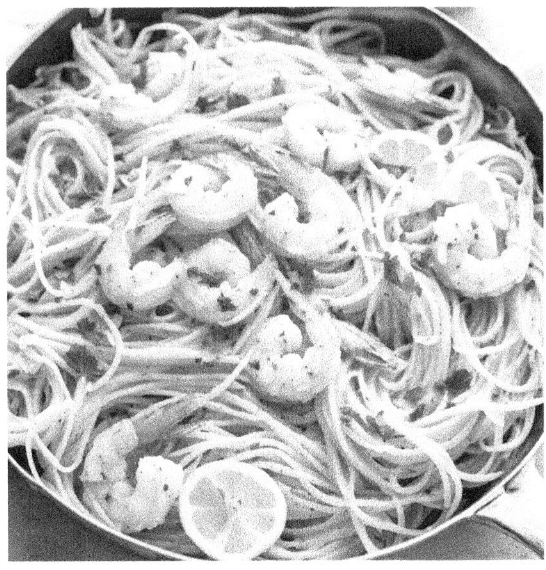

6. Mackerel Pate

Ingredients

- 2 smoked mackerel fillets, skin removed
- 1/2 cup Greek yogurt
- 1 tablespoon lemon juice
- 1 tablespoon chopped fresh dill
- 1 clove garlic, minced
- 1 teaspoon Dijon mustard

Instructions

1. In a food processor, combine the smoked mackerel, Greek yogurt, lemon juice, fresh dill, minced garlic, and Dijon mustard.
2. Process until smooth and creamy.
3. Transfer to a bowl and chill in the refrigerator for at least 1 hour before serving.
4. Serve with gluten-free crackers or vegetable sticks.

Nutrition Info per Serving

- Calories: 180
- Protein: 15g
- Fat: 10g
- Carbohydrates: 3g
- Fiber: 0g
- Sugar: 2g

Serves

4

Cooking Time

10 minutes (plus chilling time)

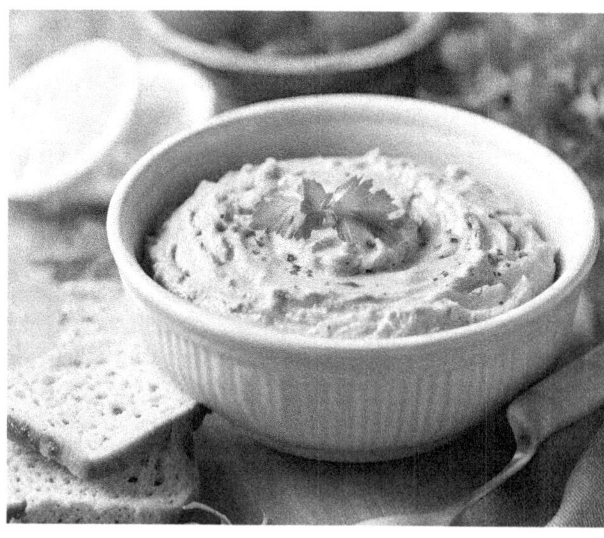

7. Clam Chowder

Ingredients

- 2 tablespoons olive oil
- 1 onion, finely chopped
- 2 cloves garlic, minced
- 2 celery stalks, diced
- 2 large potatoes, peeled and diced
- 1 can (14 ounces) chopped clams, with juice
- 4 cups vegetable broth
- 1 cup unsweetened almond milk
- 1 teaspoon dried thyme
- 1 bay leaf

Instructions

1. Heat the olive oil in a large pot over medium heat.
2. Add the onion, garlic, and celery, and sauté for about 5 minutes until softened.
3. Add the diced potatoes, chopped clams with their juice, vegetable broth, dried thyme, and bay leaf. Bring to a boil.
4. Reduce heat and simmer for about 15 minutes until the potatoes are tender.
5. Stir in the almond milk and cook for an additional 5 minutes.
6. Remove the bay leaf before serving.
7. Serve hot.

Nutrition Info per Serving

- Calories: 220
- Protein: 10g
- Fat: 8g
- Carbohydrates: 28g
- Fiber: 4g
- Sugar: 4g

Serves

4

Cooking Time

30 minutes

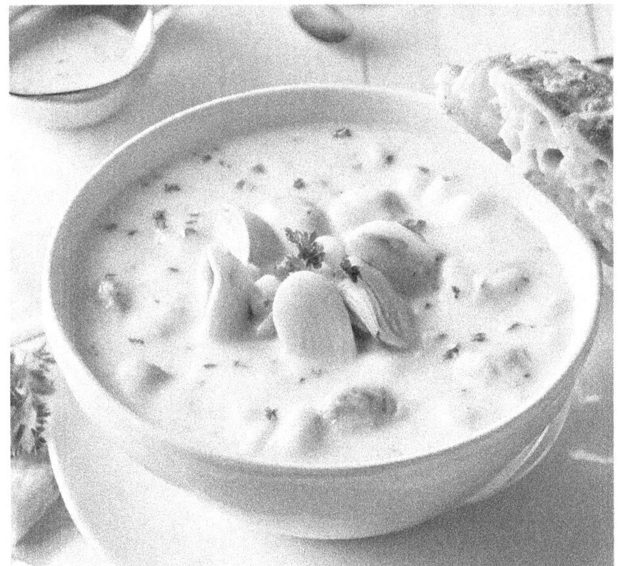

8. Grilled Trout with Almondine Sauce

Ingredients

- 4 trout fillets
- 2 tablespoons olive oil
- 1/4 cup sliced almonds
- 2 tablespoons lemon juice
- 2 tablespoons chopped fresh parsley
- 1 tablespoon olive oil

Instructions

1. Preheat the grill to medium-high heat.
2. Brush the trout fillets with 2 tablespoons of olive oil.
3. Grill the trout for about 3-4 minutes on each side until the fish flakes easily with a fork.
4. While the trout is grilling, heat 1 tablespoon of olive oil in a small skillet over medium heat.
5. Add the sliced almonds and cook for about 2-3 minutes until golden brown.
6. Remove from heat and stir in the lemon juice and chopped parsley.
7. Serve the grilled trout fillets topped with the almondine sauce.

Nutrition Info per Serving

- Calories: 300
- Protein: 25g
- Fat: 20g
- Carbohydrates: 2g
- Fiber: 1g
- Sugar: 0g

Serves

4

Cooking Time

15 minutes

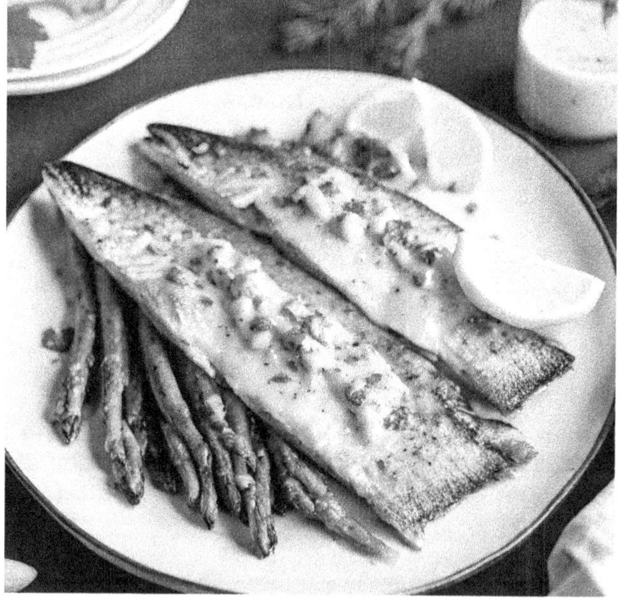

9. Crab Stuffed Mushrooms

Ingredients

- 16 large mushrooms, stems removed
- 1 can (6 ounces) crab meat, drained and flaked
- 1/4 cup Greek yogurt
- 2 tablespoons almond flour
- 2 tablespoons chopped fresh chives
- 1 tablespoon lemon juice
- 1 clove garlic, minced
- 2 tablespoons olive oil

Instructions

1. Preheat the oven to 375°F (190°C). Line a baking sheet with parchment paper.
2. In a bowl, mix the crab meat, Greek yogurt, almond flour, chopped chives, lemon juice, and minced garlic until well combined.
3. Spoon the crab mixture into the mushroom caps and place them on the prepared baking sheet.
4. Drizzle the stuffed mushrooms with olive oil.
5. Bake for about 15-20 minutes until the mushrooms are tender and the filling is golden brown.
6. Serve hot.

Nutrition Info per Serving

- Calories: 100
- Protein: 10g
- Fat: 6g
- Carbohydrates: 4g
- Fiber: 1g
- Sugar: 1g

Serves

4

Cooking Time

25 minutes

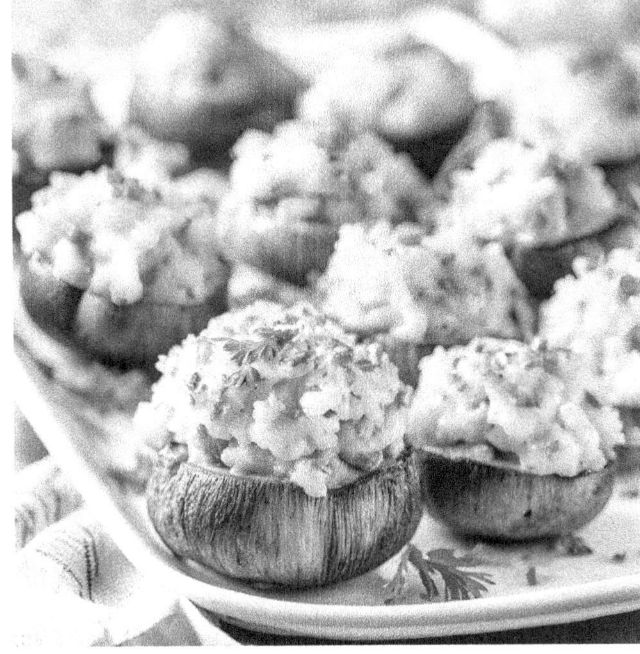

10. Baked Tilapia with Tomato Basil

Ingredients

- 4 tilapia fillets
- 2 tablespoons olive oil
- 1 pint cherry tomatoes, halved
- 2 cloves garlic, minced
- 1/4 cup fresh basil, chopped
- 1 tablespoon lemon juice

Instructions

1. Preheat the oven to 375°F (190°C).
2. Place the tilapia fillets in a baking dish and drizzle with olive oil and lemon juice.
3. Scatter the cherry tomatoes and minced garlic around the tilapia.
4. Bake for about 15-20 minutes, until the fish flakes easily with a fork.
5. Remove from the oven and sprinkle with fresh basil before serving.

Nutrition Info per Serving

- Calories: 250
- Protein: 30g
- Fat: 10g
- Carbohydrates: 8g
- Fiber: 2g
- Sugar: 4g

Serves

4

Cooking Time

25 minutes

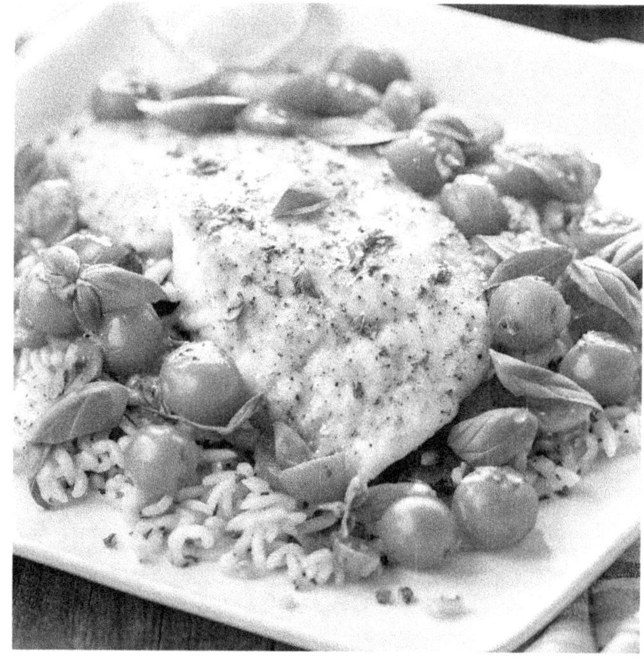

11. Cajun Catfish

Ingredients

- 4 catfish fillets
- 2 tablespoons olive oil
- 1 tablespoon Cajun seasoning
- 1 lemon, sliced

Instructions

1. Preheat the oven to 375°F (190°C).
2. Brush the catfish fillets with olive oil and sprinkle with Cajun seasoning.
3. Place the fillets on a baking sheet and top with lemon slices.
4. Bake for about 15-20 minutes, until the fish flakes easily with a fork.
5. Serve hot.

Nutrition Info per Serving

- Calories: 220
- Protein: 28g
- Fat: 11g
- Carbohydrates: 2g
- Fiber: 1g
- Sugar: 0g

Serves

4

Cooking Time

20 minutes

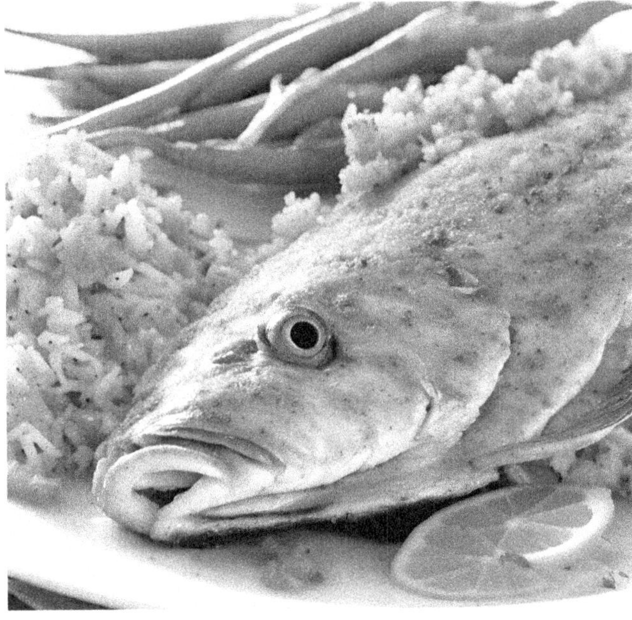

12. Sardine and Kale Pasta

Ingredients

- 8 ounces gluten-free pasta
- 2 tablespoons olive oil
- 1 can (4 ounces) sardines in olive oil, drained and flaked
- 2 cloves garlic, minced
- 1 bunch kale, stems removed and leaves chopped
- 1/4 cup lemon juice
- 1/4 cup pine nuts, toasted

Instructions

1. Cook the gluten-free pasta according to package instructions. Drain and set aside.
2. In a large skillet, heat the olive oil over medium heat.
3. Add the garlic and cook for about 1 minute until fragrant.
4. Add the chopped kale and cook for about 5 minutes until wilted.
5. Stir in the sardines and cooked pasta. Cook for an additional 2 minutes until heated through.
6. Remove from heat and stir in the lemon juice.
7. Serve topped with toasted pine nuts.

Nutrition Info per Serving

- Calories: 350
- Protein: 18g
- Fat: 16g
- Carbohydrates: 35g
- Fiber: 4g
- Sugar: 2g

Serves

4

Cooking Time

20 minutes

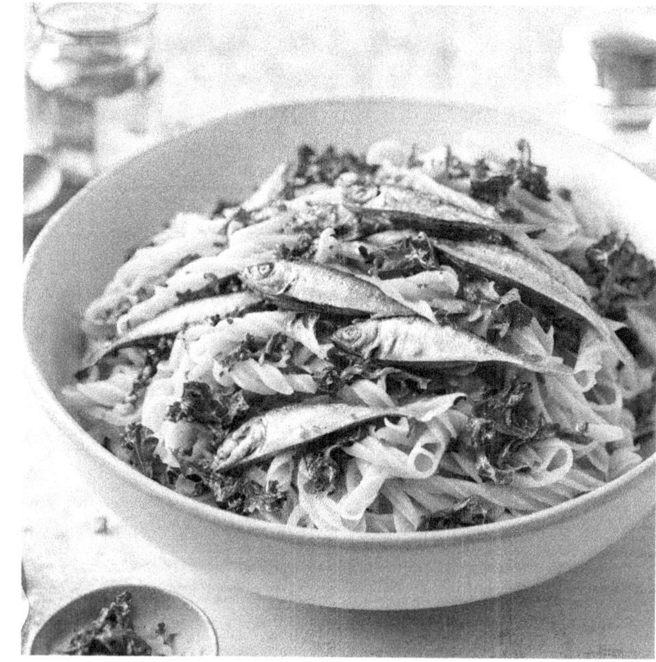

13. Fish Curry with Coconut Milk

Ingredients

- 2 tablespoons coconut oil
- 1 onion, finely chopped
- 3 cloves garlic, minced
- 1 tablespoon grated ginger
- 1 tablespoon curry powder
- 1 can (14 ounces) coconut milk
- 4 cups vegetable broth
- 1 pound white fish fillets (such as cod or tilapia), cut into chunks
- 1 red bell pepper, chopped
- 1 cup snap peas
- 2 tablespoons lime juice
- 1/4 cup fresh cilantro, chopped

Instructions

1. Heat the coconut oil in a large pot over medium heat.
2. Add the onion, garlic, and grated ginger, and sauté for about 5 minutes until softened.
3. Stir in the curry powder and cook for 2 minutes.
4. Add the coconut milk and vegetable broth. Bring to a boil, then reduce heat and simmer for about 10 minutes.
5. Add the fish chunks, red bell pepper, and snap peas. Cook for about 5-7 minutes until the fish is cooked through.
6. Remove from heat and stir in the lime juice.
7. Serve hot, garnished with fresh cilantro.

Nutrition Info per Serving

- Calories: 320
- Protein: 25g
- Fat: 20g
- Carbohydrates: 12g
- Fiber: 3g
- Sugar: 5g

Serves

4

Cooking Time

30 minutes

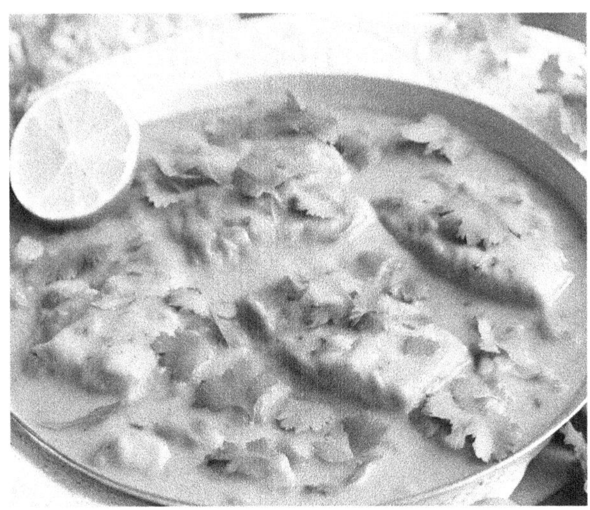

14. Haddock in Parchment with Vegetables

Ingredients

- 4 haddock fillets
- 1 zucchini, sliced
- 1 yellow squash, sliced
- 1 red bell pepper, sliced
- 2 tablespoons olive oil
- 2 tablespoons lemon juice
- 1 tablespoon fresh thyme leaves

Instructions

1. Preheat the oven to 375°F (190°C).
2. Cut four large pieces of parchment paper.
3. In the center of each piece of parchment paper, place a haddock fillet and a mix of sliced zucchini, yellow squash, and red bell pepper.
4. Drizzle each with olive oil and lemon juice, and sprinkle with fresh thyme leaves.
5. Fold the parchment paper over the fish and vegetables, and seal the edges to form a packet.
6. Place the packets on a baking sheet and bake for about 15-20 minutes, until the fish flakes easily with a fork.
7. Serve hot.

Nutrition Info per Serving

- Calories: 250
- Protein: 28g
- Fat: 12g
- Carbohydrates: 8g
- Fiber: 3g
- Sugar: 4g

Serves

4

Cooking Time

25 minutes

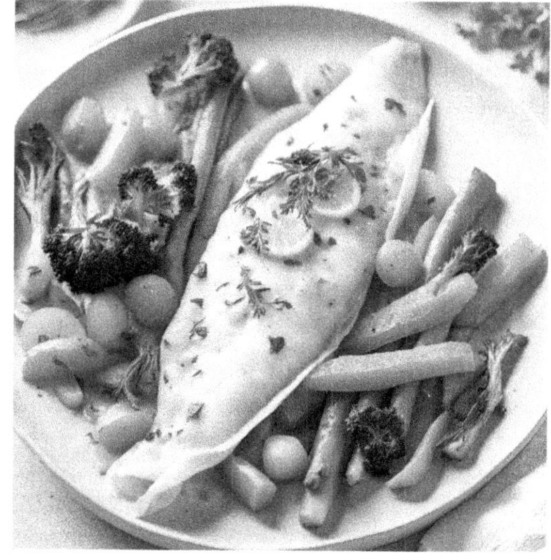

15. Smoked Salmon Frittata

Ingredients

- 8 large eggs
- 1/4 cup unsweetened almond milk
- 1 cup baby spinach, chopped
- 4 ounces smoked salmon, chopped
- 1/2 cup cherry tomatoes, halved
- 1 tablespoon olive oil
- 1/4 cup chopped fresh dill

Instructions

1. Preheat the oven to 375°F (190°C).
2. In a large bowl, whisk together the eggs and almond milk until well combined.
3. Stir in the chopped spinach, smoked salmon, cherry tomatoes, and fresh dill.
4. Heat the olive oil in an oven-safe skillet over medium heat.
5. Pour the egg mixture into the skillet and cook for about 5 minutes, until the edges start to set.
6. Transfer the skillet to the preheated oven and bake for 15-20 minutes, until the frittata is fully set and lightly browned.
7. Remove from the oven and let it cool slightly before slicing and serving.

Nutrition Info per Serving

- Calories: 200
- Protein: 18g
- Fat: 14g
- Carbohydrates: 3g
- Fiber: 1g
- Sugar: 1g

Serves

4

Cooking Time

30 minutes

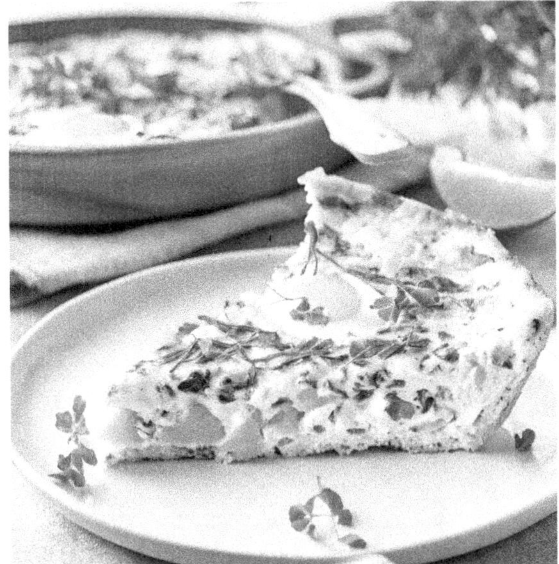

16. Garlic Butter Halibut

Ingredients

- 4 halibut fillets (about 6 ounces each)
- 3 tablespoons unsalted butter
- 4 cloves garlic, minced
- 1 tablespoon lemon juice
- 1 tablespoon chopped fresh parsley

Instructions

1. Preheat the oven to 400°F (200°C).
2. In a small saucepan, melt the butter over medium heat. Add the minced garlic and cook for 1-2 minutes until fragrant.
3. Stir in the lemon juice and remove from heat.
4. Place the halibut fillets in a baking dish and pour the garlic butter mixture over them.
5. Bake for 12-15 minutes, until the fish flakes easily with a fork.
6. Garnish with chopped parsley before serving.

Nutrition Info per Serving

- Calories: 280
- Protein: 30g
- Fat: 16g
- Carbohydrates: 1g
- Fiber: 0g
- Sugar: 0g

Serves

4

Cooking Time

20 minutes

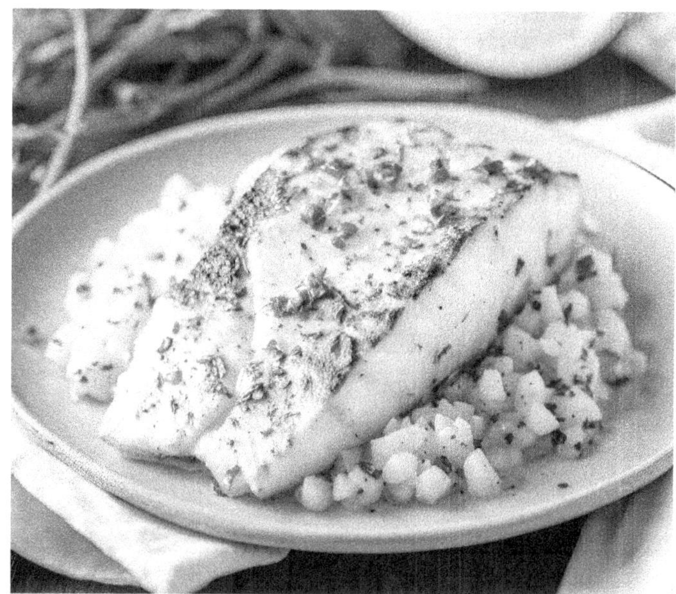

17. Shrimp and Broccoli Alfredo

Ingredients

- 8 ounces gluten-free pasta
- 1 tablespoon olive oil
- 1 pound large shrimp, peeled and deveined
- 2 cups broccoli florets
- 3 cloves garlic, minced
- 1 cup coconut milk
- 1/2 cup nutritional yeast
- 1/4 cup chopped fresh parsley

Instructions

1. Cook the gluten-free pasta according to package instructions. Drain and set aside.
2. In a large skillet, heat the olive oil over medium heat.
3. Add the shrimp and cook for about 2-3 minutes until they turn pink and are cooked through. Remove shrimp from the skillet and set aside.
4. In the same skillet, add the broccoli florets and cook for about 5 minutes until tender-crisp.
5. Add the minced garlic and cook for another 1 minute until fragrant.
6. Stir in the coconut milk and nutritional yeast. Cook for 2-3 minutes until the sauce thickens slightly.
7. Return the shrimp to the skillet and add the cooked pasta. Toss to combine and heat through.
8. Serve garnished with chopped parsley.

Nutrition Info per Serving

- Calories: 400
- Protein: 28g
- Fat: 14g
- Carbohydrates: 40g
- Fiber: 6g
- Sugar: 3g

Serves

4

Cooking Time

20 minutes

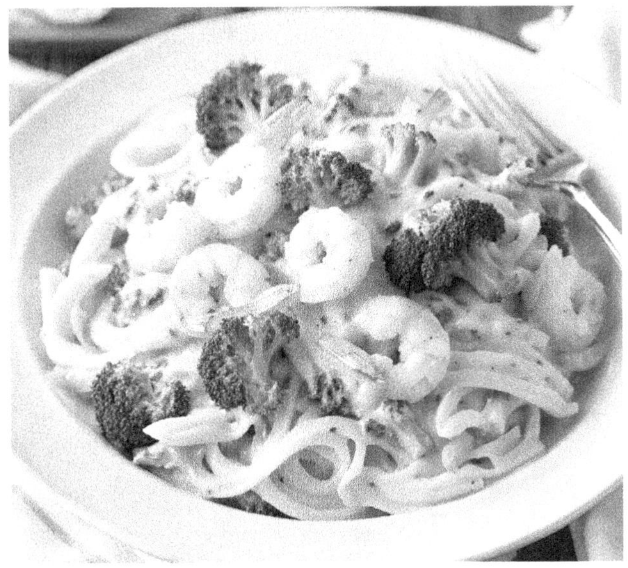

18. Peppered Tuna Steak

Ingredients

- 4 tuna steaks (about 6 ounces each)
- 2 tablespoons olive oil
- 2 teaspoons coarsely ground black pepper
- 1 tablespoon lemon juice

Instructions

1. Preheat a grill or grill pan to medium-high heat.
2. Brush the tuna steaks with olive oil and sprinkle with coarsely ground black pepper.
3. Grill the tuna steaks for about 2-3 minutes on each side, until they are cooked to your desired doneness.
4. Drizzle with lemon juice before serving.

Nutrition Info per Serving

- Calories: 250
- Protein: 34g
- Fat: 12g
- Carbohydrates: 0g
- Fiber: 0g
- Sugar: 0g

Serves

4

Cooking Time

10 minutes

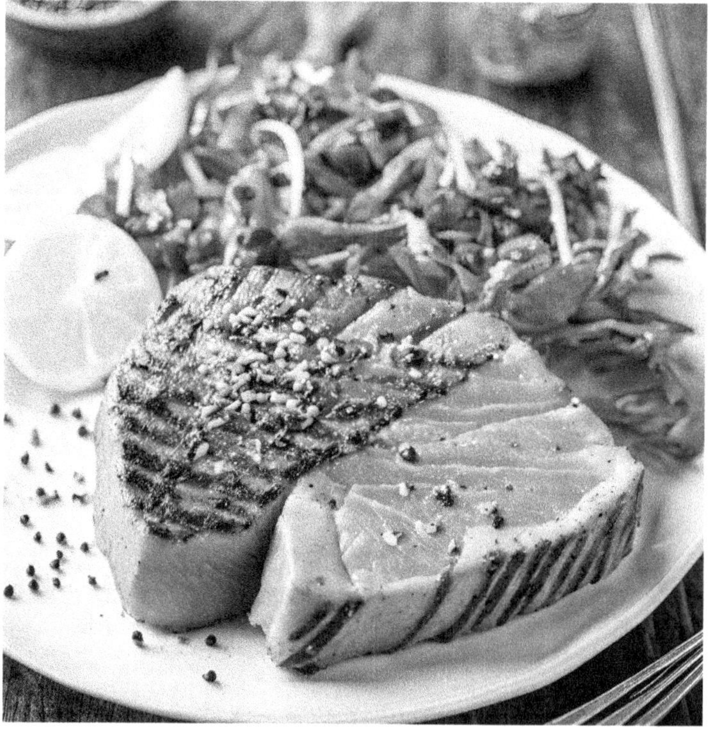

19. Sea Bass with Citrus Salsa

Ingredients

- 4 sea bass fillets (about 6 ounces each)
- 2 tablespoons olive oil
- 1 orange, peeled and diced
- 1 grapefruit, peeled and diced
- 1/4 cup red onion, finely chopped
- 1/4 cup fresh cilantro, chopped
- 1 tablespoon lime juice

Instructions

1. Preheat the oven to 375°F (190°C).
2. Brush the sea bass fillets with olive oil and place them on a baking sheet.
3. Bake for 15-20 minutes, until the fish flakes easily with a fork.
4. While the fish is baking, prepare the citrus salsa. In a bowl, combine the diced orange, grapefruit, red onion, fresh cilantro, and lime juice.
5. Serve the baked sea bass topped with the citrus salsa.

Nutrition Info per Serving

- Calories: 300
- Protein: 30g
- Fat: 12g
- Carbohydrates: 12g
- Fiber: 2g
- Sugar: 8g

Serves

4

Cooking Time

25 minutes

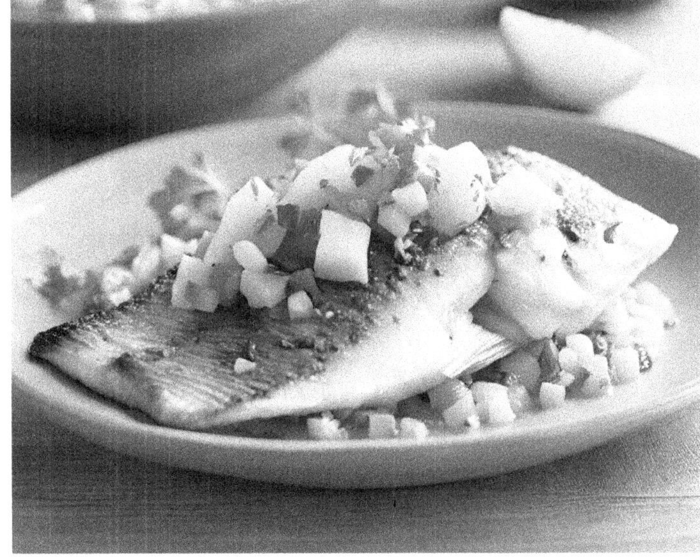

20. Anchovy and Tomato Salad

Ingredients

- 1 pint cherry tomatoes, halved
- 1/4 cup red onion, finely chopped
- 1/4 cup Kalamata olives, pitted and halved
- 8 anchovy fillets, chopped
- 2 tablespoons olive oil
- 1 tablespoon red wine vinegar
- 1 tablespoon fresh basil, chopped

Instructions

1. In a large bowl, combine the cherry tomatoes, red onion, Kalamata olives, and chopped anchovy fillets.
2. In a small bowl, whisk together the olive oil and red wine vinegar.
3. Pour the dressing over the salad and toss to combine.
4. Garnish with fresh basil.
5. Serve immediately.

Nutrition Info per Serving

- Calories: 160
- Protein: 6g
- Fat: 12g
- Carbohydrates: 8g
- Fiber: 2g
- Sugar: 4g

Serves

4

Cooking Time

10 minutes

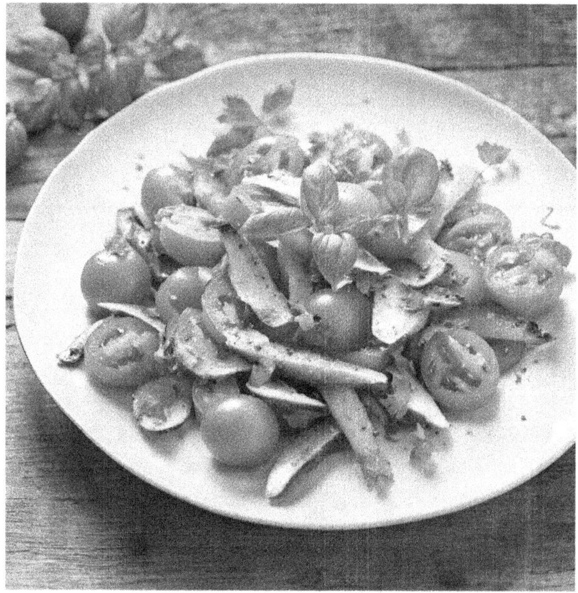

21. Barramundi with Lemon Caper Sauce

Ingredients

- 4 barramundi fillets (about 6 ounces each)
- 2 tablespoons olive oil
- 1/4 cup capers, drained
- 1/4 cup lemon juice
- 1 tablespoon chopped fresh parsley
- 2 cloves garlic, minced

Instructions

1. Preheat the oven to 375°F (190°C).
2. Brush the barramundi fillets with 1 tablespoon of olive oil and place them on a baking sheet.
3. Bake for 15-20 minutes, until the fish flakes easily with a fork.
4. While the fish is baking, heat the remaining olive oil in a small skillet over medium heat.
5. Add the capers and garlic, and cook for 2-3 minutes until the garlic is fragrant.
6. Stir in the lemon juice and cook for another 2 minutes.
7. Remove from heat and stir in the chopped parsley.
8. Serve the barramundi fillets topped with the lemon caper sauce.

Nutrition Info per Serving

- Calories: 260
- Protein: 32g
- Fat: 12g
- Carbohydrates: 3g
- Fiber: 1g
- Sugar: 1g

Serves

4

Cooking Time

25 minutes

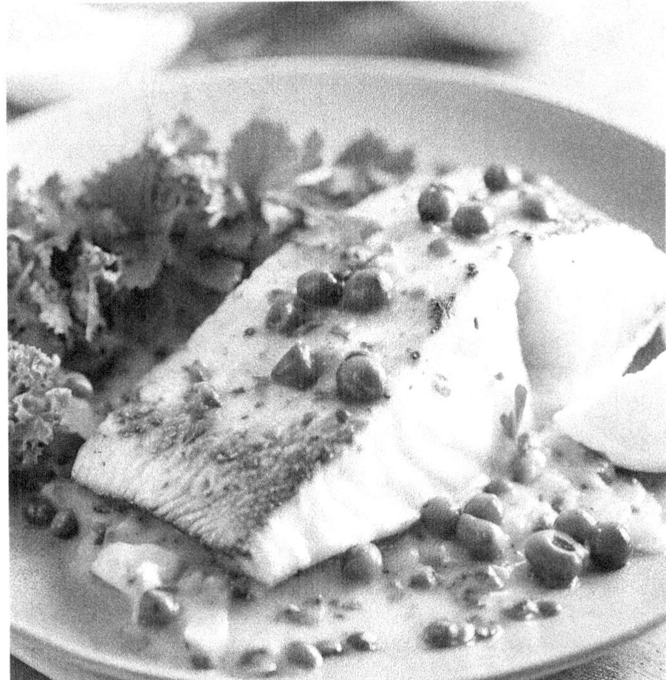

22. Cod and Asparagus Bake

Ingredients

- 4 cod fillets (about 6 ounces each)
- 1 pound asparagus, trimmed
- 2 tablespoons olive oil
- 1 tablespoon lemon juice
- 1 teaspoon dried thyme
- 1/4 cup grated Parmesan cheese (optional)

Instructions

1. Preheat the oven to 400°F (200°C).
2. Arrange the cod fillets and asparagus in a baking dish.
3. Drizzle with olive oil and lemon juice.
4. Sprinkle with dried thyme and grated Parmesan cheese (if using).
5. Bake for 15-20 minutes, until the fish flakes easily with a fork and the asparagus is tender.
6. Serve hot.

Nutrition Info per Serving

- Calories: 220
- Protein: 30g
- Fat: 10g
- Carbohydrates: 5g
- Fiber: 2g
- Sugar: 2g

Serves
4

Cooking Time
20 minutes

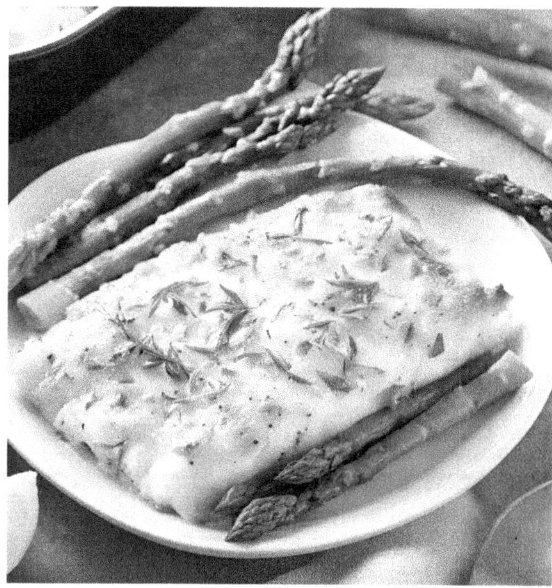

23. Shrimp Gazpacho

Ingredients

- 1 pound large shrimp, peeled, deveined, and cooked
- 4 large tomatoes, diced
- 1 cucumber, peeled and diced
- 1 red bell pepper, diced
- 1/4 cup red onion, finely chopped
- 2 cloves garlic, minced
- 2 cups tomato juice
- 1/4 cup olive oil
- 2 tablespoons red wine vinegar
- 1 tablespoon fresh cilantro, chopped

Instructions

1. In a large bowl, combine the diced tomatoes, cucumber, red bell pepper, red onion, garlic, and cooked shrimp.
2. Stir in the tomato juice, olive oil, and red wine vinegar.
3. Chill the soup in the refrigerator for at least 1 hour before serving.
4. Garnish with fresh cilantro.
5. Serve cold.

Nutrition Info per Serving

- Calories: 220
- Protein: 22g
- Fat: 12g
- Carbohydrates: 10g
- Fiber: 3g
- Sugar: 6g

Serves

4

Cooking Time

15 minutes (plus chilling time)

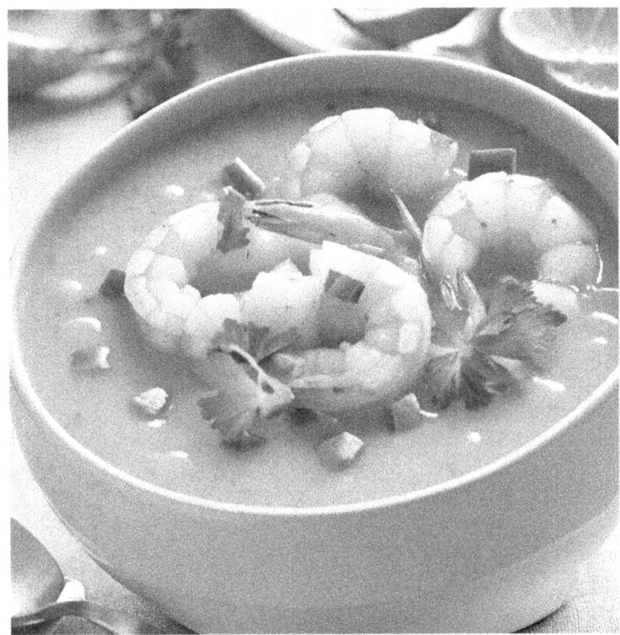

24. Scallops with Ginger Soy Glaze

Ingredients

- 1 pound large scallops
- 2 tablespoons olive oil
- 1 tablespoon grated fresh ginger
- 2 cloves garlic, minced
- 1/4 cup tamari (gluten-free soy sauce)
- 1 tablespoon honey
- 1 tablespoon lime juice
- 1 tablespoon chopped fresh cilantro

Instructions

1. Pat the scallops dry with paper towels.
2. Heat the olive oil in a large skillet over medium-high heat.
3. Add the scallops and sear for about 2-3 minutes on each side until golden brown and cooked through. Remove from the skillet and set aside.
4. In the same skillet, add the grated ginger and minced garlic. Cook for about 1 minute until fragrant.
5. Stir in the tamari, honey, and lime juice. Cook for another 2 minutes until the sauce thickens slightly.
6. Return the scallops to the skillet and coat them with the sauce.
7. Serve garnished with fresh cilantro.

Nutrition Info per Serving

- Calories: 210
- Protein: 24g
- Fat: 8g
- Carbohydrates: 10g
- Fiber: 0g
- Sugar: 6g

Serves

4

Cooking Time

15 minutes

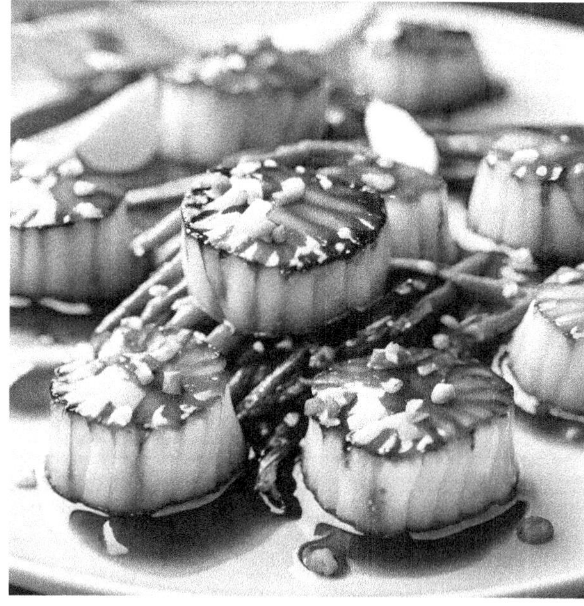

Poultry Recipes

1. Grilled Chicken with Avocado Salsa

Ingredients

- 4 boneless, skinless chicken breasts
- 2 tablespoons olive oil
- 1 teaspoon ground cumin
- 1 teaspoon garlic powder
- 1 avocado, diced
- 1 cup cherry tomatoes, halved
- 1/4 cup red onion, finely chopped
- 1 tablespoon lime juice
- 2 tablespoons fresh cilantro, chopped

Instructions

1. Preheat the grill to medium-high heat.
2. In a small bowl, mix the olive oil, ground cumin, and garlic powder. Brush the mixture over the chicken breasts.
3. Grill the chicken for about 6-7 minutes on each side, or until the internal temperature reaches 165°F (74°C) and the chicken is cooked through.
4. While the chicken is grilling, prepare the avocado salsa. In a medium bowl, combine the diced avocado, cherry tomatoes, red onion, lime juice, and fresh cilantro.
5. Serve the grilled chicken breasts topped with the avocado salsa.

Nutrition Info per Serving

- Calories: 320
- Protein: 30g
- Fat: 20g
- Carbohydrates: 8g
- Fiber: 4g
- Sugar: 2g

Serves

4

Cooking Time

20 minutes

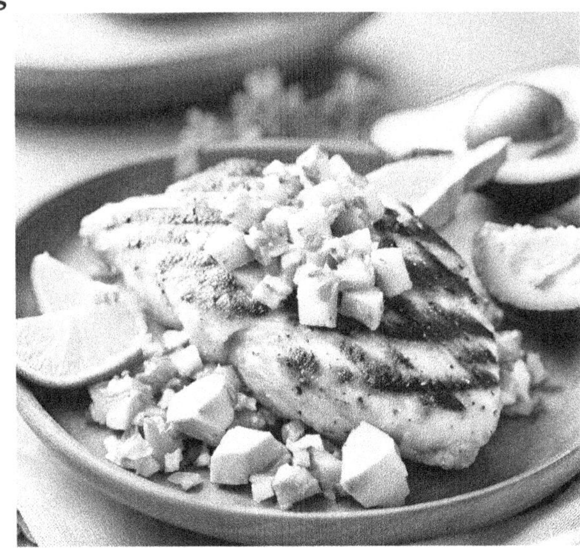

2. Turmeric Turkey Wraps

Ingredients

- 1 pound ground turkey
- 1 tablespoon olive oil
- 1 teaspoon ground turmeric
- 1 teaspoon ground cumin
- 1/2 teaspoon garlic powder
- 1/4 cup chopped fresh parsley
- 4 large lettuce leaves (for wraps)
- 1 avocado, sliced
- 1/2 cup shredded carrots

Instructions

1. In a large skillet, heat the olive oil over medium heat.
2. Add the ground turkey, turmeric, cumin, and garlic powder. Cook for about 8-10 minutes, breaking up the turkey with a spatula, until fully cooked.
3. Stir in the chopped parsley.
4. Lay the lettuce leaves flat and fill each with the cooked turkey mixture.
5. Top with sliced avocado and shredded carrots.
6. Roll up the lettuce leaves to form wraps and serve.

Nutrition Info per Serving

- Calories: 250
- Protein: 22g
- Fat: 15g
- Carbohydrates: 6g
- Fiber: 3g
- Sugar: 2g

Serves

4

Cooking Time

15 minutes

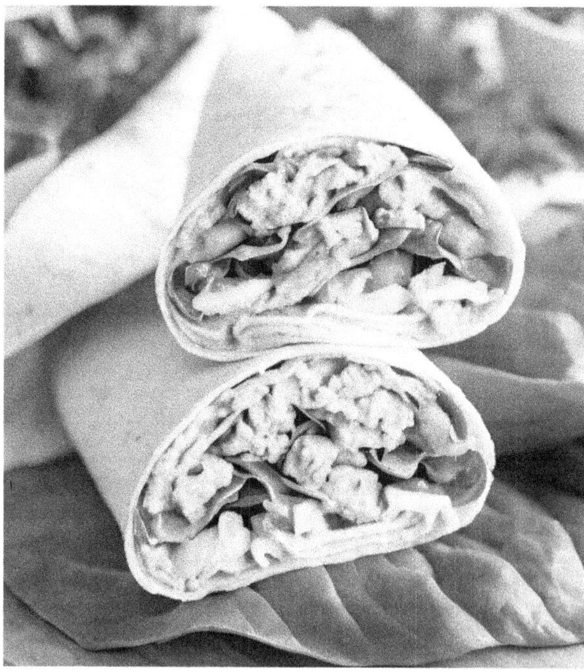

3. Chicken and Spinach Stew

Ingredients

- 1 tablespoon olive oil
- 1 onion, finely chopped
- 2 cloves garlic, minced
- 1 pound boneless, skinless chicken thighs, cut into chunks
- 4 cups chicken broth
- 2 large potatoes, peeled and diced
- 1 teaspoon ground cumin
- 1 teaspoon ground coriander
- 4 cups fresh spinach, chopped

Instructions

1. Heat the olive oil in a large pot over medium heat.
2. Add the onion and garlic, and sauté for about 5 minutes until softened.
3. Add the chicken thighs and cook for about 5-7 minutes until browned on all sides.
4. Stir in the chicken broth, diced potatoes, cumin, and coriander. Bring to a boil.
5. Reduce heat and simmer for about 20 minutes until the potatoes are tender and the chicken is cooked through.
6. Stir in the chopped spinach and cook for an additional 5 minutes until wilted.
7. Serve hot.

Nutrition Info per Serving

- Calories: 320
- Protein: 30g
- Fat: 12g
- Carbohydrates: 22g
- Fiber: 4g
- Sugar: 2g

Serves

4

Cooking Time

40 minutes

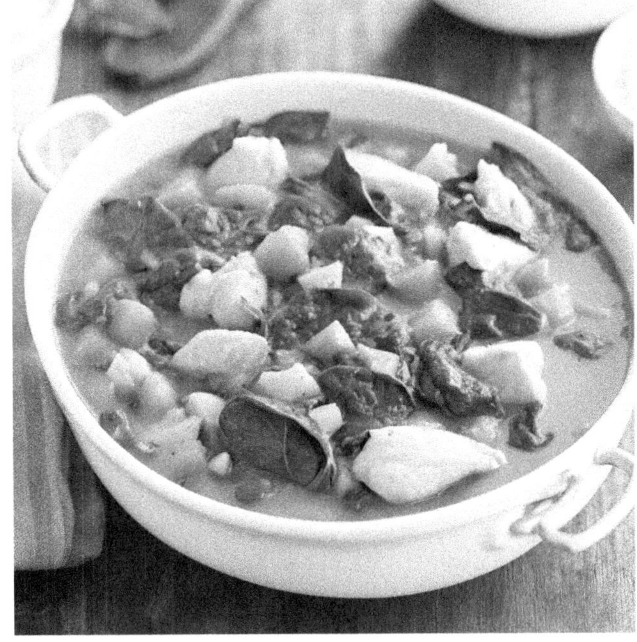

4. Turkey Quinoa Meatballs

Ingredients

- 1 pound ground turkey
- 1/2 cup cooked quinoa
- 1/4 cup finely chopped onion
- 2 cloves garlic, minced
- 1 tablespoon ground flaxseed
- 1 teaspoon dried oregano
- 1 egg, beaten
- 1 tablespoon olive oil

Instructions

1. Preheat the oven to 375°F (190°C). Line a baking sheet with parchment paper.
2. In a large bowl, combine the ground turkey, cooked quinoa, chopped onion, minced garlic, ground flaxseed, dried oregano, and beaten egg. Mix until well combined.
3. Form the mixture into small meatballs and place them on the prepared baking sheet.
4. Brush the meatballs with olive oil.
5. Bake for 20-25 minutes, until the meatballs are cooked through and lightly browned.
6. Serve hot.

Nutrition Info per Serving

- Calories: 200
- Protein: 25g
- Fat: 8g
- Carbohydrates: 8g
- Fiber: 1g
- Sugar: 1g

Serves

4

Cooking Time

30 minutes

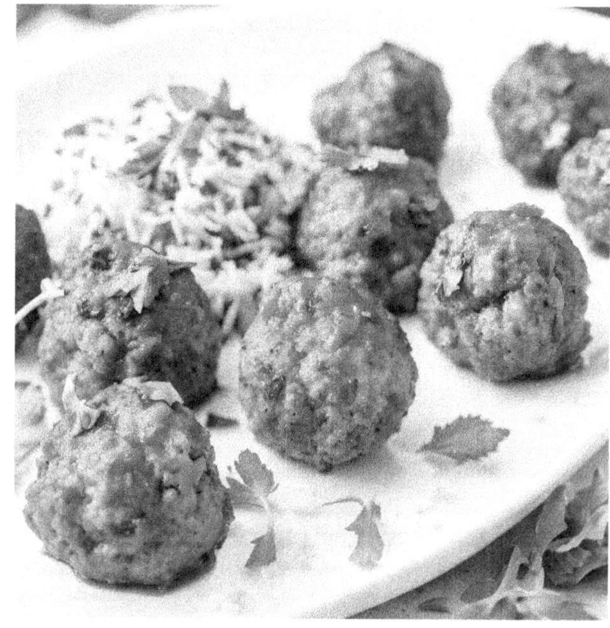

5. Chicken Ginger Soup

Ingredients

- 1 tablespoon olive oil
- 1 onion, finely chopped
- 3 cloves garlic, minced
- 1 tablespoon grated fresh ginger
- 1 pound boneless, skinless chicken breasts, cut into thin strips
- 6 cups chicken broth
- 2 carrots, sliced
- 2 celery stalks, sliced
- 1 cup sliced mushrooms
- 1 cup baby spinach
- 2 tablespoons lime juice
- 1/4 cup fresh cilantro, chopped

Instructions

1. Heat the olive oil in a large pot over medium heat.
2. Add the onion, garlic, and grated ginger, and sauté for about 5 minutes until softened.
3. Add the chicken strips and cook for about 5 minutes until browned.
4. Stir in the chicken broth, carrots, celery, and mushrooms. Bring to a boil.
5. Reduce heat and simmer for about 15 minutes until the vegetables are tender and the chicken is cooked through.
6. Stir in the baby spinach and cook for an additional 2 minutes until wilted.
7. Remove from heat and stir in the lime juice.
8. Serve hot, garnished with fresh cilantro.

Nutrition Info per Serving

- Calories: 220
- Protein: 30g
- Fat: 6g
- Carbohydrates: 14g
- Fiber: 3g
- Sugar: 5g

Serves

4

Cooking Time

30 minutes

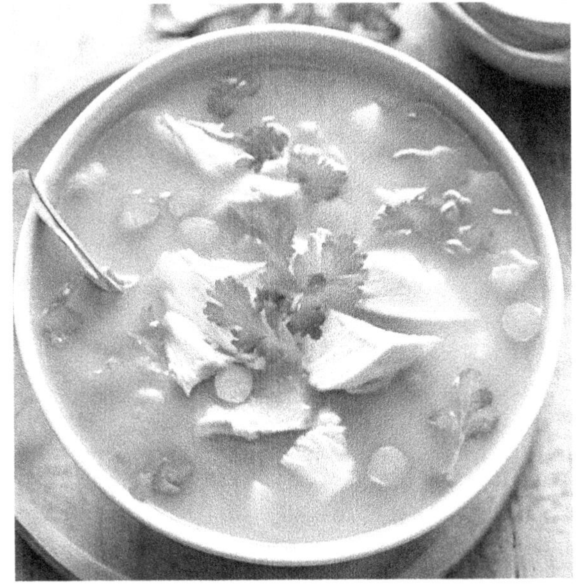

6. Cilantro Lime Chicken Skewers

Ingredients

- 1 pound boneless, skinless chicken breasts, cut into cubes
- 2 tablespoons olive oil
- 2 tablespoons lime juice
- 2 cloves garlic, minced
- 1/4 cup fresh cilantro, chopped
- 1 teaspoon ground cumin

Instructions

1. In a large bowl, mix the olive oil, lime juice, minced garlic, chopped cilantro, and ground cumin.
2. Add the chicken cubes and toss to coat evenly. Marinate in the refrigerator for at least 30 minutes.
3. Preheat the grill to medium-high heat.
4. Thread the marinated chicken onto skewers.
5. Grill the chicken skewers for about 5-7 minutes on each side, until fully cooked.
6. Serve hot.

Nutrition Info per Serving

- Calories: 190
- Protein: 28g
- Fat: 8g
- Carbohydrates: 2g
- Fiber: 1g
- Sugar: 0g

Serves

4

Cooking Time

15 minutes (plus marinating time)

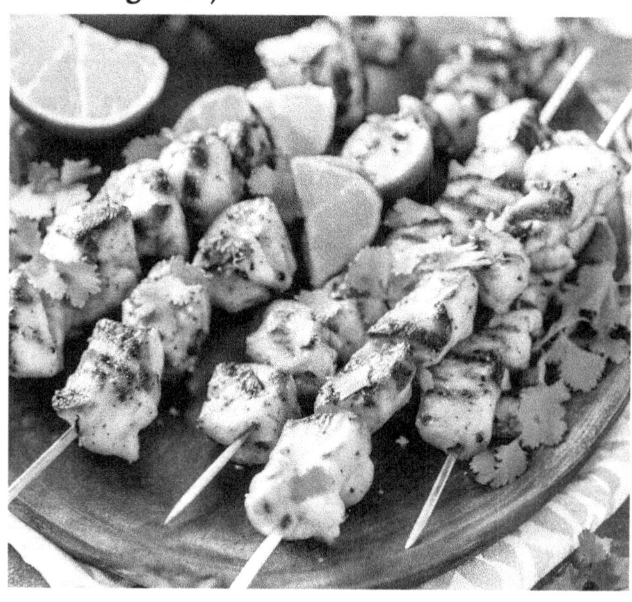

7. Turkey Stuffed Peppers

Ingredients

- 4 large bell peppers
- 1 pound ground turkey
- 1 tablespoon olive oil
- 1 onion, finely chopped
- 2 cloves garlic, minced
- 1 cup cooked quinoa
- 1 can (14 ounces) diced tomatoes, drained
- 1 teaspoon dried oregano
- 1 teaspoon ground cumin
- 1/4 cup chopped fresh parsley

Instructions

1. Preheat the oven to 375°F (190°C).
2. Cut the tops off the bell peppers and remove the seeds and membranes. Place the peppers in a baking dish.
3. In a large skillet, heat the olive oil over medium heat.
4. Add the onion and garlic, and sauté for about 5 minutes until softened.
5. Add the ground turkey, oregano, and cumin, and cook for about 8-10 minutes until the turkey is fully cooked.
6. Stir in the cooked quinoa and diced tomatoes. Cook for an additional 5 minutes.
7. Stuff the bell peppers with the turkey mixture and place in the baking dish.
8. Cover the dish with foil and bake for 30 minutes.
9. Remove the foil and bake for an additional 10 minutes.
10. Garnish with chopped fresh parsley before serving.

Nutrition Info per Serving

- Calories: 280
- Protein: 25g
- Fat: 10g
- Carbohydrates: 22g
- Fiber: 5g
- Sugar: 8g

Serves

4

Cooking Time

50 minutes

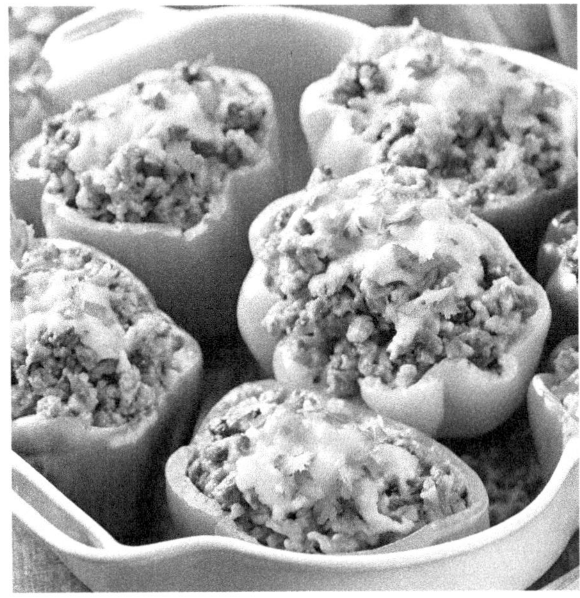

8. Rosemary Chicken Salad

Ingredients

- 1 pound boneless, skinless chicken breasts
- 2 tablespoons olive oil
- 2 teaspoons dried rosemary
- 4 cups mixed salad greens
- 1/2 cup cherry tomatoes, halved
- 1/4 cup red onion, thinly sliced
- 1/4 cup walnuts, chopped
- 1 avocado, sliced
- 1 tablespoon balsamic vinegar

Instructions

1. Preheat the oven to 375°F (190°C).
2. Rub the chicken breasts with olive oil and sprinkle with dried rosemary.
3. Place the chicken on a baking sheet and bake for 25-30 minutes, until fully cooked.
4. Allow the chicken to cool slightly, then slice into strips.
5. In a large bowl, combine the salad greens, cherry tomatoes, red onion, walnuts, and avocado.
6. Add the sliced chicken on top.
7. Drizzle with balsamic vinegar before serving.

Nutrition Info per Serving

- Calories: 300
- Protein: 28g
- Fat: 18g
- Carbohydrates: 10g
- Fiber: 5g
- Sugar: 3g

Serves

4

Cooking Time

30 minutes

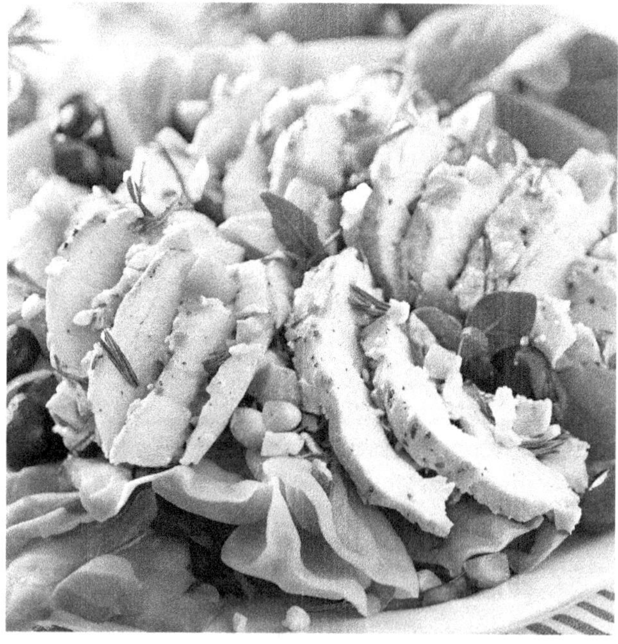

9. Smoky Turkey Chili

Ingredients

- 1 tablespoon olive oil
- 1 onion, finely chopped
- 2 cloves garlic, minced
- 1 pound ground turkey
- 1 teaspoon ground cumin
- 1 teaspoon smoked paprika
- 1/2 teaspoon ground coriander
- 1 can (14 ounces) diced tomatoes
- 1 can (15 ounces) black beans, drained and rinsed
- 1 cup vegetable broth
- 1/4 cup chopped fresh cilantro

Instructions

1. In a large pot, heat the olive oil over medium heat.
2. Add the onion and garlic, and sauté for about 5 minutes until softened.
3. Add the ground turkey, cumin, smoked paprika, and coriander. Cook for about 8-10 minutes, breaking up the turkey with a spatula, until fully cooked.
4. Stir in the diced tomatoes, black beans, and vegetable broth. Bring to a boil.
5. Reduce heat and simmer for about 20 minutes until the flavors are well combined.
6. Serve hot, garnished with chopped fresh cilantro.

Nutrition Info per Serving

- Calories: 280
- Protein: 25g
- Fat: 10g
- Carbohydrates: 22g
- Fiber: 6g
- Sugar: 5g

Serves

4

Cooking Time

35 minutes

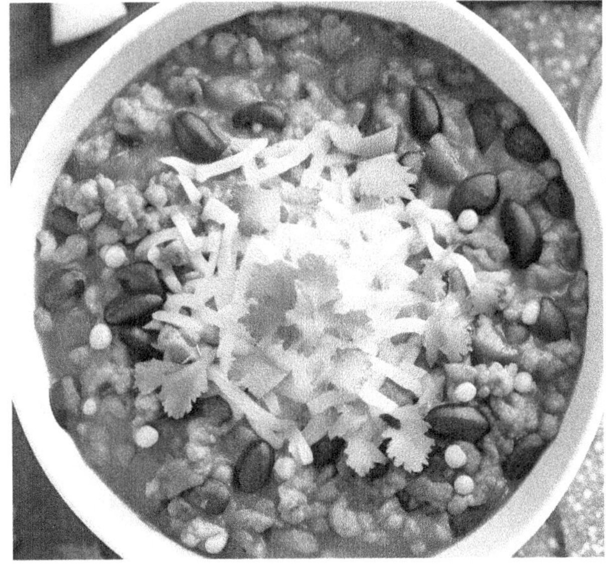

10. Turkey and Sweet Potato Skillet
Ingredients
- 1 pound ground turkey
- 2 tablespoons olive oil
- 1 onion, finely chopped
- 2 cloves garlic, minced
- 2 large sweet potatoes, peeled and diced
- 1 teaspoon ground cumin
- 1 teaspoon smoked paprika
- 2 cups baby spinach
- 1 tablespoon fresh parsley, chopped

Instructions
1. In a large skillet, heat the olive oil over medium heat.
2. Add the onion and garlic, and sauté for about 5 minutes until softened.
3. Add the ground turkey and cook for about 8-10 minutes until fully cooked.
4. Stir in the diced sweet potatoes, ground cumin, and smoked paprika. Cook for about 15 minutes until the sweet potatoes are tender.
5. Stir in the baby spinach and cook for an additional 2 minutes until wilted.
6. Garnish with fresh parsley and serve hot.

Nutrition Info per Serving
- Calories: 320
- Protein: 25g
- Fat: 14g
- Carbohydrates: 28g
- Fiber: 5g
- Sugar: 7g

Serves
4
Cooking Time
30 minutes

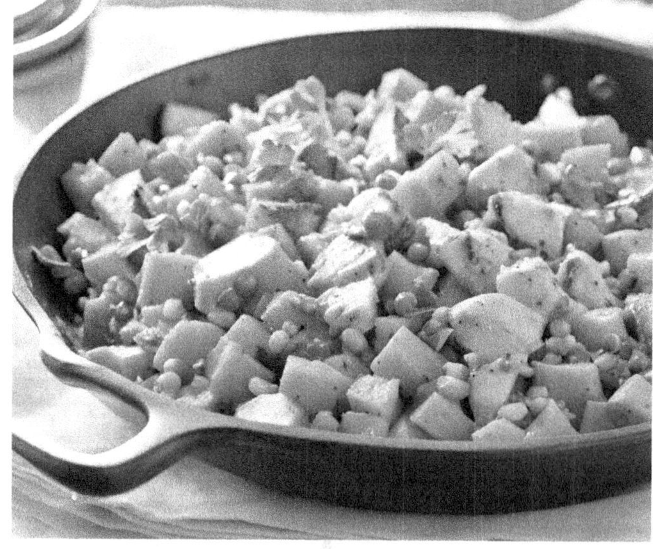

11. Lemon Herb Roasted Chicken

Ingredients

- 1 whole chicken (about 4 pounds)
- 4 tablespoons olive oil
- 2 tablespoons lemon juice
- 1 tablespoon dried oregano
- 1 tablespoon dried thyme
- 1 lemon, sliced
- 4 cloves garlic, minced
- 1/4 cup fresh parsley, chopped

Instructions

1. Preheat the oven to 375°F (190°C).
2. In a small bowl, mix the olive oil, lemon juice, dried oregano, dried thyme, and minced garlic.
3. Rub the mixture all over the chicken, making sure to coat it evenly.
4. Place the lemon slices inside the chicken cavity.
5. Place the chicken on a roasting pan and roast for about 1 hour and 20 minutes, or until the internal temperature reaches 165°F (74°C).
6. Remove from the oven and let the chicken rest for 10 minutes before carving.
7. Garnish with fresh parsley and serve.

Nutrition Info per Serving

- Calories: 450
- Protein: 35g
- Fat: 32g
- Carbohydrates: 3g
- Fiber: 1g
- Sugar: 1g

Serves

6

Cooking Time

1 hour 30 minutes

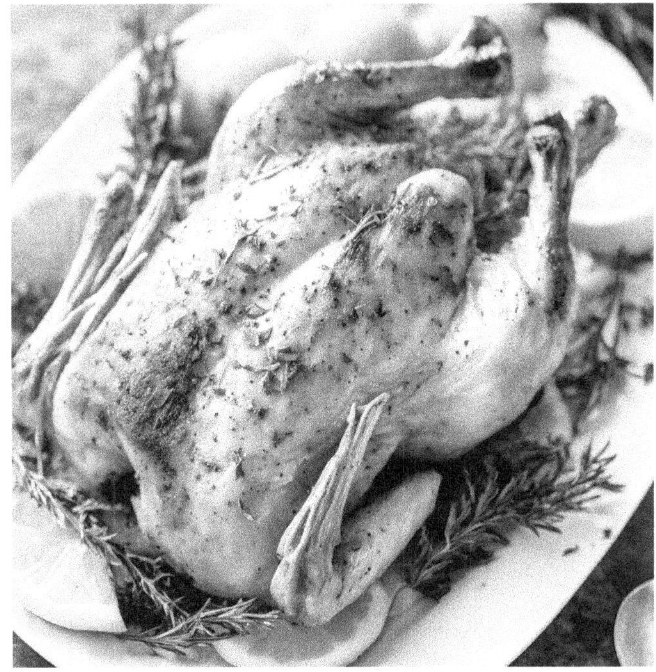

12. Chicken and Broccoli Alfredo

Ingredients

- 8 ounces gluten-free pasta
- 1 tablespoon olive oil
- 1 pound boneless, skinless chicken breasts, cut into strips
- 3 cloves garlic, minced
- 2 cups broccoli florets
- 1 cup coconut milk
- 1/2 cup nutritional yeast
- 1/4 cup fresh parsley, chopped

Instructions

1. Cook the gluten-free pasta according to package instructions. Drain and set aside.
2. In a large skillet, heat the olive oil over medium heat.
3. Add the chicken strips and cook for about 6-7 minutes until fully cooked. Remove from the skillet and set aside.
4. In the same skillet, add the minced garlic and cook for about 1 minute until fragrant.
5. Add the broccoli florets and cook for about 5 minutes until tender-crisp.
6. Stir in the coconut milk and nutritional yeast. Cook for about 2-3 minutes until the sauce thickens.
7. Return the chicken to the skillet and add the cooked pasta. Toss to combine and heat through.
8. Garnish with fresh parsley and serve hot.

Nutrition Info per Serving

- Calories: 350
- Protein: 28g
- Fat: 14g
- Carbohydrates: 32g
- Fiber: 5g
- Sugar: 3g

Serves

4

Cooking Time

25 minutes

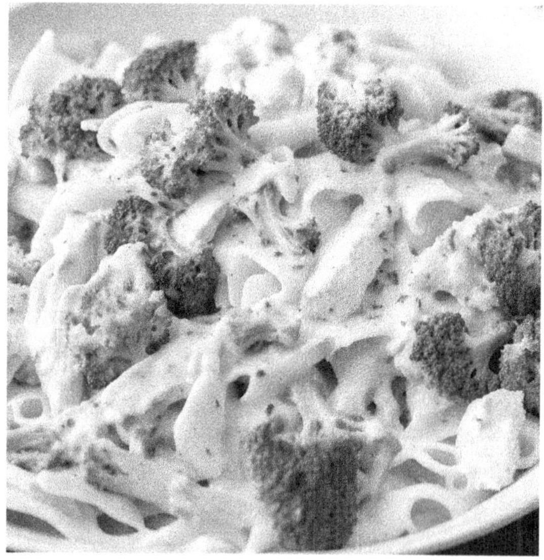

13. Balsamic Glazed Turkey Breast

Ingredients

- 1 pound turkey breast
- 2 tablespoons olive oil
- 1/4 cup balsamic vinegar
- 2 tablespoons honey
- 1 teaspoon dried thyme
- 3 cloves garlic, minced

Instructions

1. Preheat the oven to 375°F (190°C).
2. In a small bowl, mix the olive oil, balsamic vinegar, honey, dried thyme, and minced garlic.
3. Place the turkey breast in a baking dish and brush with the balsamic mixture.
4. Bake for about 30-35 minutes, or until the internal temperature reaches 165°F (74°C), basting occasionally with the glaze.
5. Remove from the oven and let rest for 10 minutes before slicing.
6. Serve hot.

Nutrition Info per Serving

- Calories: 280
- Protein: 28g
- Fat: 10g
- Carbohydrates: 20g
- Fiber: 1g
- Sugar: 18g

Serves

4

Cooking Time

40 minutes

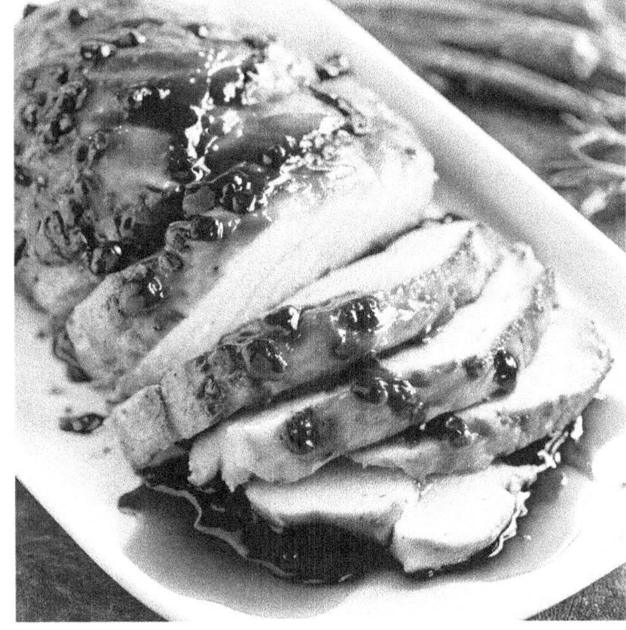

14. Chicken Cauliflower Fried Rice

Ingredients

- 1 head cauliflower, grated or processed into rice-sized pieces
- 2 tablespoons olive oil
- 1 pound boneless, skinless chicken breasts, diced
- 2 cloves garlic, minced
- 1 cup frozen peas and carrots, thawed
- 2 eggs, beaten
- 2 tablespoons tamari (gluten-free soy sauce)
- 1 tablespoon sesame oil
- 1/4 cup green onions, chopped

Instructions

1. In a large skillet, heat 1 tablespoon of olive oil over medium heat.
2. Add the diced chicken and cook for about 5-7 minutes until fully cooked. Remove from the skillet and set aside.
3. In the same skillet, heat the remaining olive oil and add the minced garlic. Cook for about 1 minute until fragrant.
4. Add the cauliflower rice and cook for about 5 minutes until tender.
5. Stir in the peas and carrots and cook for another 2 minutes.
6. Push the cauliflower mixture to the side of the skillet and pour the beaten eggs into the empty side. Scramble the eggs until fully cooked, then mix with the cauliflower rice.
7. Return the chicken to the skillet and stir in the tamari and sesame oil. Cook for another 2 minutes until heated through.
8. Garnish with chopped green onions and serve hot.

Nutrition Info per Serving

- Calories: 320
- Protein: 28g
- Fat: 18g
- Carbohydrates: 12g
- Fiber: 4g
- Sugar: 4g

Serves

4

Cooking Time

20 minutes

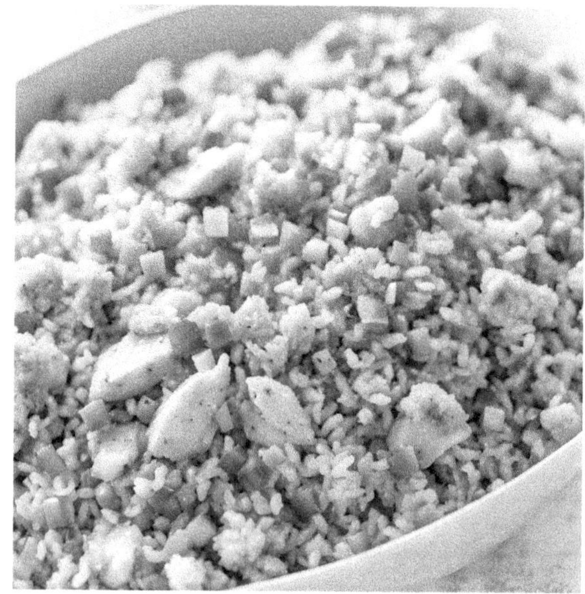

15. Buffalo Turkey Meatballs

Ingredients

- 1 pound ground turkey
- 1/4 cup almond flour
- 1 egg, beaten
- 2 cloves garlic, minced
- 1 teaspoon dried parsley
- 1/2 cup hot sauce (such as Frank's RedHot)
- 2 tablespoons unsalted butter, melted

Instructions

1. Preheat the oven to 375°F (190°C). Line a baking sheet with parchment paper.
2. In a large bowl, mix the ground turkey, almond flour, beaten egg, minced garlic, and dried parsley until well combined.
3. Form the mixture into small meatballs and place them on the prepared baking sheet.
4. Bake for 20-25 minutes, until the meatballs are cooked through.
5. While the meatballs are baking, mix the hot sauce and melted butter in a small bowl.
6. Toss the cooked meatballs in the buffalo sauce until evenly coated.
7. Serve hot.

Nutrition Info per Serving

- Calories: 200
- Protein: 20g
- Fat: 12g
- Carbohydrates: 3g
- Fiber: 1g
- Sugar: 1g

Serves

4

Cooking Time

30 minutes

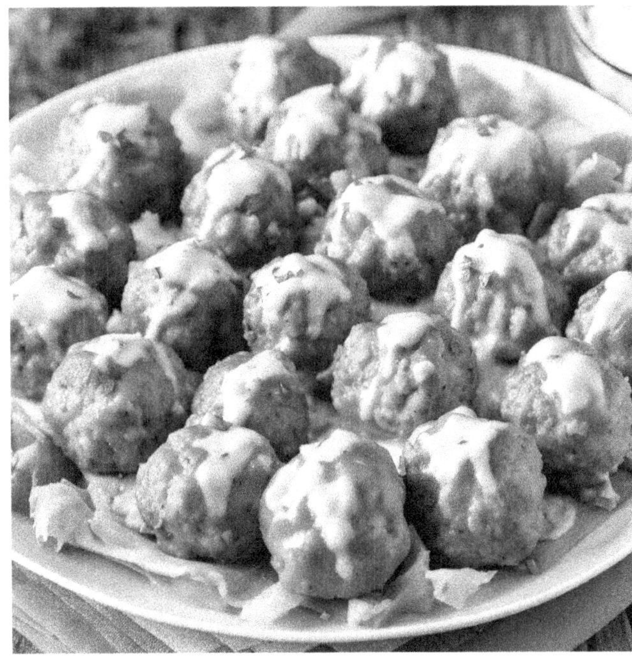

16. Mediterranean Turkey Meatloaf

Ingredients

- 1 pound ground turkey
- 1/2 cup cooked quinoa
- 1/4 cup sun-dried tomatoes, chopped
- 1/4 cup Kalamata olives, pitted and chopped
- 2 cloves garlic, minced
- 1 egg, beaten
- 1 tablespoon dried oregano
- 1/4 cup crumbled feta cheese (optional)

Instructions

1. Preheat the oven to 375°F (190°C). Line a loaf pan with parchment paper.
2. In a large bowl, mix the ground turkey, cooked quinoa, sun-dried tomatoes, Kalamata olives, minced garlic, beaten egg, dried oregano, and feta cheese (if using) until well combined.
3. Press the mixture into the prepared loaf pan.
4. Bake for 45-50 minutes, until the meatloaf is cooked through and a meat thermometer reads 165°F (74°C).
5. Let the meatloaf rest for 10 minutes before slicing.
6. Serve hot.

Nutrition Info per Serving

- Calories: 250
- Protein: 22g
- Fat: 12g
- Carbohydrates: 12g
- Fiber: 3g
- Sugar: 3g

Serves

4

Cooking Time

50 minutes

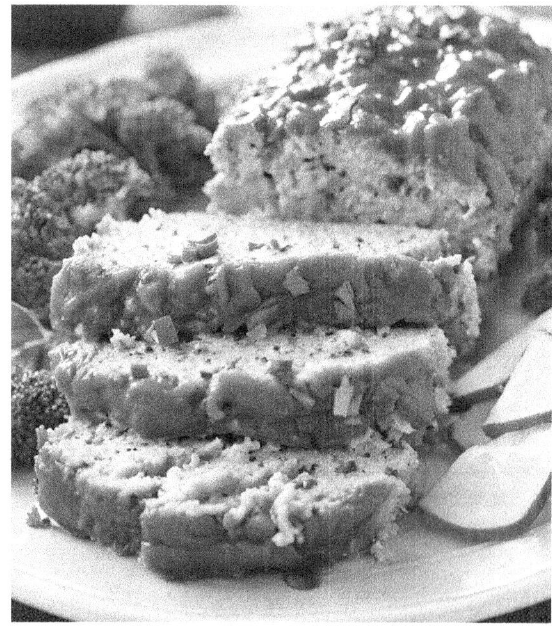

17. Chicken Zoodle Soup

Ingredients

- 1 tablespoon olive oil
- 1 onion, finely chopped
- 2 cloves garlic, minced
- 2 carrots, sliced
- 2 celery stalks, sliced
- 1 pound boneless, skinless chicken breasts, cut into cubes
- 6 cups chicken broth
- 2 medium zucchinis, spiralized into zoodles
- 1 teaspoon dried thyme
- 1 teaspoon dried basil

Instructions

1. Heat the olive oil in a large pot over medium heat.
2. Add the onion, garlic, carrots, and celery, and sauté for about 5 minutes until softened.
3. Add the chicken cubes and cook for about 5 minutes until browned on all sides.
4. Stir in the chicken broth, dried thyme, and dried basil. Bring to a boil.
5. Reduce heat and simmer for about 15 minutes until the chicken is cooked through and the vegetables are tender.
6. Stir in the zucchini noodles and cook for an additional 2 minutes until tender.
7. Serve hot.

Nutrition Info per Serving

- Calories: 200
- Protein: 25g
- Fat: 7g
- Carbohydrates: 12g
- Fiber: 3g
- Sugar: 5g

Serves

4

Cooking Time

30 minutes

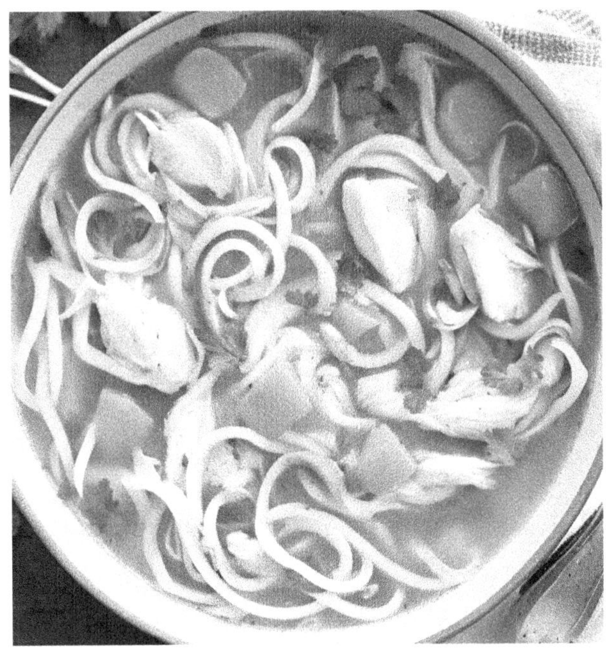

18. Herb Roasted Turkey Thighs

Ingredients

- 4 turkey thighs
- 2 tablespoons olive oil
- 1 tablespoon dried rosemary
- 1 tablespoon dried thyme
- 4 cloves garlic, minced
- 1 lemon, sliced

Instructions

1. Preheat the oven to 375°F (190°C). Line a baking dish with parchment paper.
2. In a small bowl, mix the olive oil, dried rosemary, dried thyme, and minced garlic.
3. Rub the mixture all over the turkey thighs, making sure to coat them evenly.
4. Arrange the lemon slices in the baking dish and place the turkey thighs on top.
5. Roast for about 1 hour and 15 minutes, or until the internal temperature reaches 165°F (74°C).
6. Let the turkey rest for 10 minutes before serving.
7. Serve hot.

Nutrition Info per Serving

- Calories: 350
- Protein: 28g
- Fat: 24g
- Carbohydrates: 2g
- Fiber: 1g
- Sugar: 1g

Serves

4

Cooking Time

1 hour 30 minutes

19. Chicken Ratatouille
Ingredients
- 1 tablespoon olive oil
- 1 onion, finely chopped
- 2 cloves garlic, minced
- 1 eggplant, diced
- 1 zucchini, diced
- 1 red bell pepper, diced
- 1 yellow bell pepper, diced
- 1 pound boneless, skinless chicken breasts, cut into cubes
- 1 can (14 ounces) diced tomatoes
- 1 teaspoon dried oregano
- 1 teaspoon dried basil

Instructions
1. Heat the olive oil in a large skillet over medium heat.
2. Add the onion and garlic, and sauté for about 5 minutes until softened.
3. Add the chicken cubes and cook for about 5 minutes until browned on all sides.
4. Stir in the eggplant, zucchini, red bell pepper, and yellow bell pepper. Cook for about 10 minutes until the vegetables are tender.
5. Add the diced tomatoes, dried oregano, and dried basil. Cook for an additional 10 minutes until the chicken is cooked through and the flavors are well combined.
6. Serve hot.

Nutrition Info per Serving
- Calories: 250
- Protein: 25g
- Fat: 10g
- Carbohydrates: 18g
- Fiber: 5g
- Sugar: 10g

Serves
4

Cooking Time
30 minutes

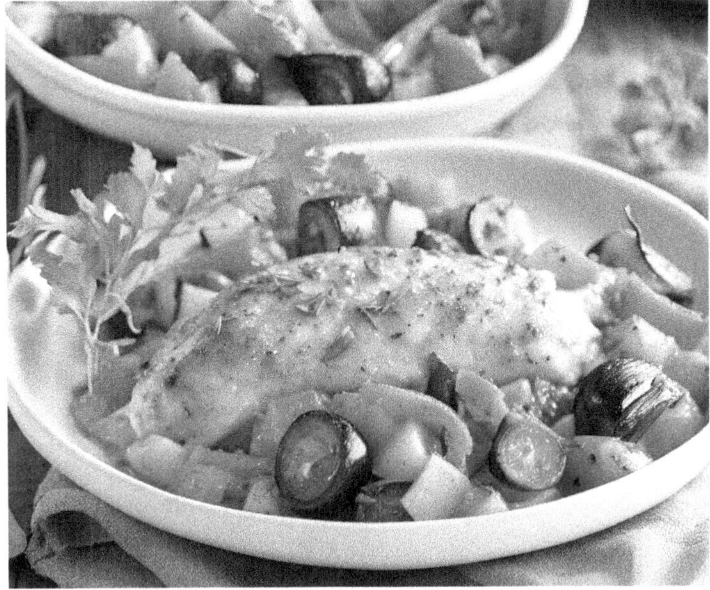

20. Stuffed Turkey Breast with Spinach and Walnuts

Ingredients

- 1 pound turkey breast, butterflied
- 2 tablespoons olive oil
- 2 cups fresh spinach, chopped
- 1/4 cup walnuts, chopped
- 1/4 cup crumbled feta cheese (optional)
- 2 cloves garlic, minced
- 1 teaspoon dried thyme

Instructions

1. Preheat the oven to 375°F (190°C).
2. In a skillet, heat 1 tablespoon of olive oil over medium heat. Add the minced garlic and cook for 1 minute until fragrant.
3. Add the spinach and cook for 2-3 minutes until wilted.
4. Stir in the chopped walnuts and feta cheese (if using).
5. Lay the butterflied turkey breast flat and spread the spinach mixture over it. Roll up the turkey breast and secure with toothpicks or kitchen twine.
6. Rub the rolled turkey breast with the remaining olive oil and sprinkle with dried thyme.
7. Place the turkey breast in a baking dish and bake for 30-35 minutes, until the internal temperature reaches 165°F (74°C).
8. Let the turkey rest for 10 minutes before slicing.
9. Serve hot.

Nutrition Info per Serving

- Calories: 300
- Protein: 28g
- Fat: 18g
- Carbohydrates: 5g
- Fiber: 2g
- Sugar: 1g

Serves

4

Cooking Time

45 minutes

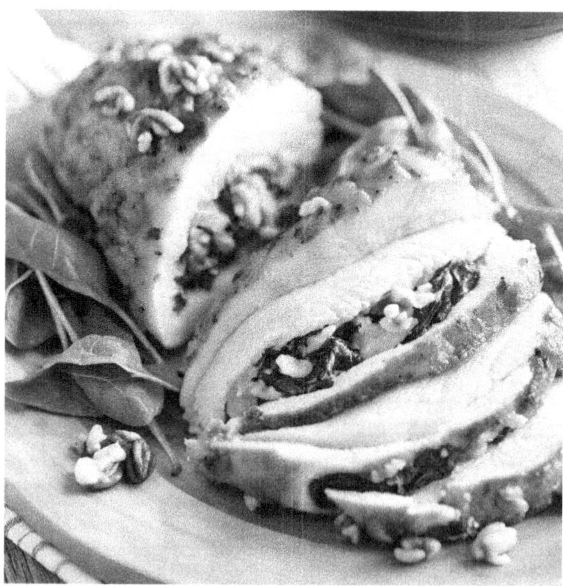

21. Chicken and Asparagus Stir-Fry

Ingredients

- 1 pound boneless, skinless chicken breasts, sliced thinly
- 2 tablespoons olive oil
- 2 cloves garlic, minced
- 1 tablespoon grated fresh ginger
- 1 bunch asparagus, trimmed and cut into 2-inch pieces
- 1 red bell pepper, sliced
- 2 tablespoons tamari (gluten-free soy sauce)
- 1 tablespoon sesame oil

Instructions

1. Heat 1 tablespoon of olive oil in a large skillet or wok over medium-high heat.
2. Add the sliced chicken and cook for about 5-7 minutes until fully cooked. Remove from the skillet and set aside.
3. In the same skillet, add the remaining olive oil, garlic, and ginger. Cook for about 1 minute until fragrant.
4. Add the asparagus and red bell pepper. Stir-fry for about 5 minutes until tender-crisp.
5. Return the chicken to the skillet and stir in the tamari and sesame oil. Cook for an additional 2 minutes until heated through.
6. Serve hot.

Nutrition Info per Serving

- Calories: 220
- Protein: 28g
- Fat: 10g
- Carbohydrates: 8g
- Fiber: 3g
- Sugar: 3g

Serves

4

Cooking Time

20 minutes

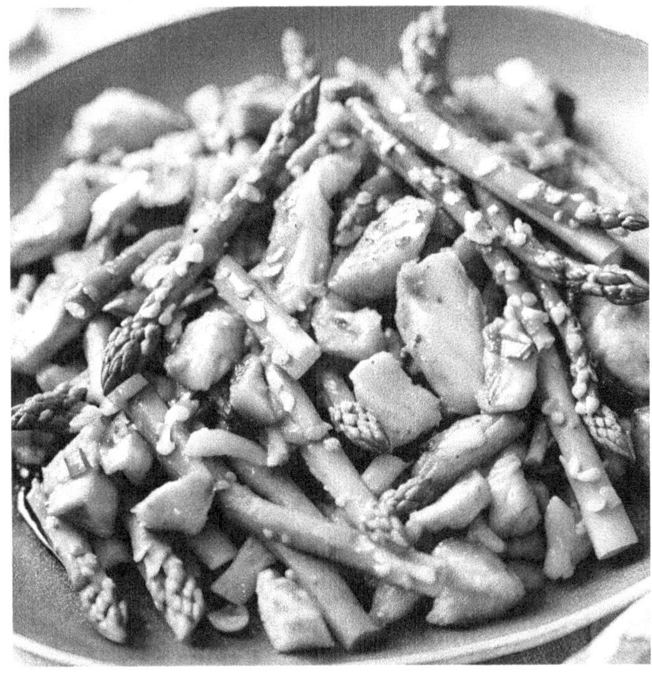

22. Turkey and Cranberry Salad

Ingredients

- 1 pound cooked turkey breast, cubed
- 1/4 cup dried cranberries
- 1/4 cup walnuts, chopped
- 1/4 cup celery, diced
- 1/4 cup Greek yogurt
- 1 tablespoon Dijon mustard
- 2 tablespoons fresh parsley, chopped

Instructions

1. In a large bowl, combine the cubed turkey, dried cranberries, chopped walnuts, and diced celery.
2. In a small bowl, mix the Greek yogurt and Dijon mustard.
3. Pour the yogurt mixture over the turkey mixture and toss to coat evenly.
4. Garnish with fresh parsley.
5. Serve immediately or chill in the refrigerator until ready to serve.

Nutrition Info per Serving

- Calories: 250
- Protein: 28g
- Fat: 10g
- Carbohydrates: 12g
- Fiber: 2g
- Sugar: 7g

Serves

4

Cooking Time

10 minutes

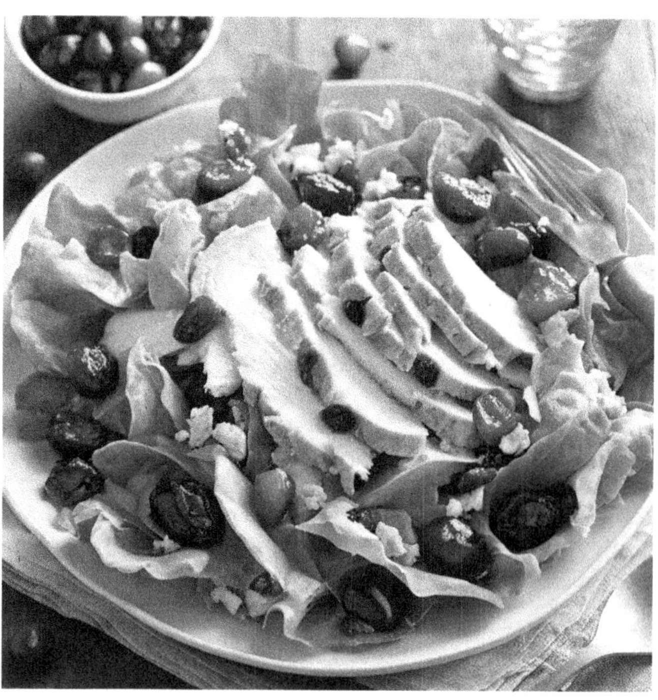

23. Chicken and Mango Chutney Sandwiches

Ingredients

- 1 pound cooked chicken breast, shredded
- 1/4 cup mango chutney
- 1/4 cup Greek yogurt
- 1 tablespoon Dijon mustard
- 4 whole grain or gluten-free sandwich rolls
- 1 cup arugula or mixed greens

Instructions

1. In a large bowl, combine the shredded chicken, mango chutney, Greek yogurt, and Dijon mustard.
2. Slice the sandwich rolls in half and toast if desired.
3. Spread the chicken mixture on the bottom halves of the rolls.
4. Top with arugula or mixed greens.
5. Place the top halves of the rolls on the sandwiches.
6. Serve immediately.

Nutrition Info per Serving

- Calories: 320
- Protein: 28g
- Fat: 8g
- Carbohydrates: 34g
- Fiber: 5g
- Sugar: 10g

Serves

4

Cooking Time

15 minutes

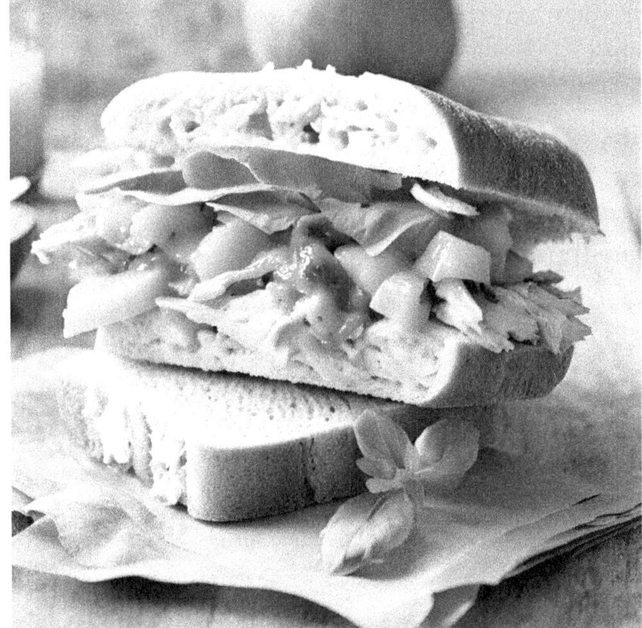

24. Turkey Veggie Meatloaf

Ingredients

- 1 pound ground turkey
- 1/2 cup cooked quinoa
- 1/2 cup grated carrots
- 1/2 cup grated zucchini
- 1 onion, finely chopped
- 2 cloves garlic, minced
- 1 egg, beaten
- 1 tablespoon dried oregano
- 1/4 cup tomato paste

Instructions

1. Preheat the oven to 375°F (190°C). Line a loaf pan with parchment paper.
2. In a large bowl, combine the ground turkey, cooked quinoa, grated carrots, grated zucchini, chopped onion, minced garlic, beaten egg, and dried oregano. Mix until well combined.
3. Press the mixture into the prepared loaf pan.
4. Spread the tomato paste evenly over the top of the meatloaf.
5. Bake for 45-50 minutes, until the meatloaf is cooked through and a meat thermometer reads 165°F (74°C).
6. Let the meatloaf rest for 10 minutes before slicing.
7. Serve hot.

Nutrition Info per Serving

- Calories: 280
- Protein: 25g
- Fat: 10g
- Carbohydrates: 20g
- Fiber: 4g
- Sugar: 6g

Serves

4

Cooking Time

50 minutes

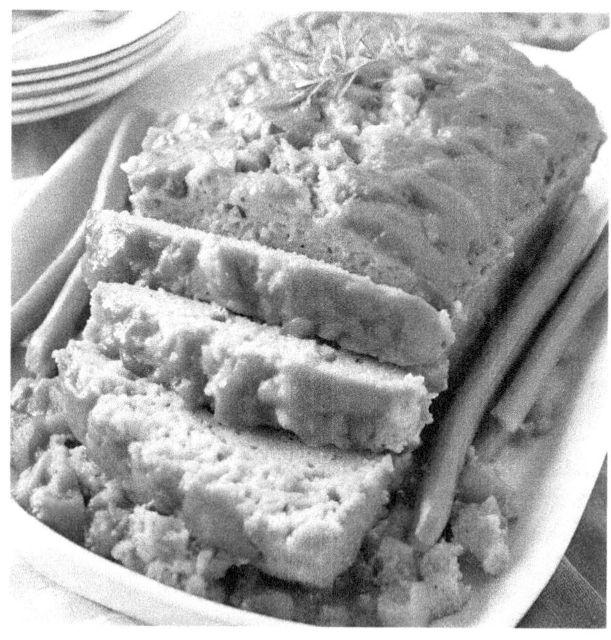

25. Garlic and Lemon Roasted Chicken Thighs

Ingredients

- 8 chicken thighs, bone-in, skin-on
- 4 tablespoons olive oil
- 4 cloves garlic, minced
- 2 tablespoons lemon juice
- 1 tablespoon dried rosemary
- 1 lemon, sliced

Instructions

1. Preheat the oven to 375°F (190°C). Line a baking dish with parchment paper.
2. In a small bowl, mix the olive oil, minced garlic, lemon juice, and dried rosemary.
3. Rub the mixture all over the chicken thighs, making sure to coat them evenly.
4. Arrange the lemon slices in the baking dish and place the chicken thighs on top.
5. Roast for about 1 hour, or until the internal temperature reaches 165°F (74°C).
6. Let the chicken rest for 10 minutes before serving.
7. Serve hot.

Nutrition Info per Serving

- Calories: 380
- Protein: 25g
- Fat: 30g
- Carbohydrates: 3g
- Fiber: 1g
- Sugar: 1g

Serves

4

Cooking Time

1 hour

Vegetables

1. Kale and Quinoa Salad
Ingredients
- 1 cup quinoa, rinsed
- 2 cups water
- 4 cups kale, chopped
- 1/4 cup dried cranberries
- 1/4 cup walnuts, chopped
- 1/4 cup feta cheese, crumbled (optional)
- 1/4 cup olive oil
- 2 tablespoons lemon juice
- 1 tablespoon Dijon mustard
- 1 garlic clove, minced

Instructions
1. In a medium saucepan, bring the water to a boil. Add the quinoa, reduce heat to low, cover, and simmer for 15 minutes or until the quinoa is tender and water is absorbed. Remove from heat and let cool.
2. In a large bowl, combine the chopped kale, cooked quinoa, dried cranberries, walnuts, and feta cheese (if using).
3. In a small bowl, whisk together the olive oil, lemon juice, Dijon mustard, and minced garlic.
4. Pour the dressing over the salad and toss to combine.
5. Serve immediately or refrigerate until ready to serve.

Nutrition Info per Serving
- Calories: 250
- Protein: 7g
- Fat: 16g
- Carbohydrates: 23g
- Fiber: 4g
- Sugar: 5g

Serves
4

Cooking Time
20 minutes

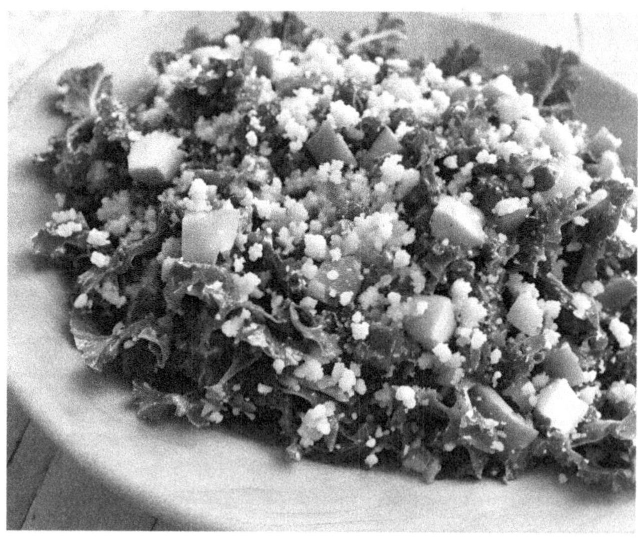

2. Turkey Soup with Kale and White Beans

Ingredients

- 1 tablespoon olive oil
- 1 onion, finely chopped
- 2 cloves garlic, minced
- 1 pound ground turkey
- 4 cups chicken broth
- 1 can (15 ounces) white beans, drained and rinsed
- 4 cups kale, chopped
- 1 teaspoon dried thyme
- 1 teaspoon dried rosemary

Instructions

1. In a large pot, heat the olive oil over medium heat. Add the onion and garlic, and sauté for about 5 minutes until softened.
2. Add the ground turkey and cook for about 8-10 minutes until browned.
3. Stir in the chicken broth, white beans, chopped kale, thyme, and rosemary. Bring to a boil.
4. Reduce heat and simmer for about 15 minutes until the kale is tender.
5. Serve hot.

Nutrition Info per Serving

- Calories: 250
- Protein: 25g
- Fat: 10g
- Carbohydrates: 18g
- Fiber: 5g
- Sugar: 2g

Serves

4

Cooking Time

30 minutes

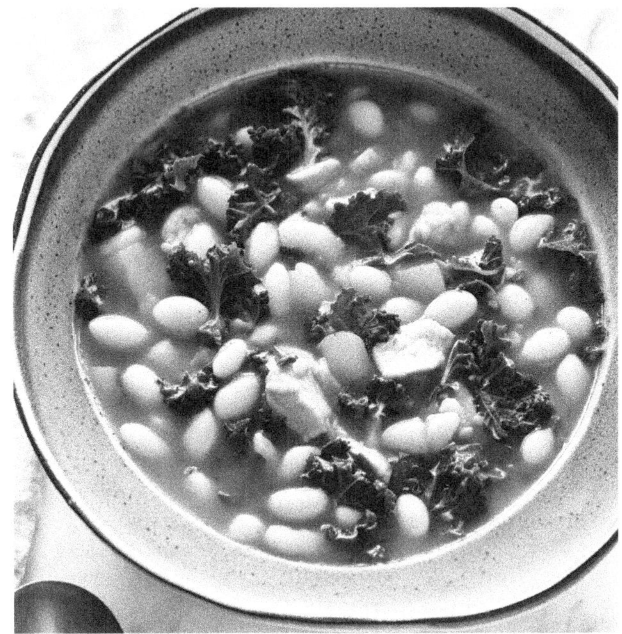

3. Sweet Potato and Ginger Soup

Ingredients

- 1 tablespoon olive oil
- 1 onion, finely chopped
- 2 cloves garlic, minced
- 1 tablespoon grated fresh ginger
- 4 cups sweet potatoes, peeled and diced
- 4 cups vegetable broth
- 1 teaspoon ground cumin
- 1 teaspoon ground coriander
- 1 cup coconut milk

Instructions

1. In a large pot, heat the olive oil over medium heat. Add the onion, garlic, and grated ginger, and sauté for about 5 minutes until softened.
2. Add the diced sweet potatoes, vegetable broth, ground cumin, and ground coriander. Bring to a boil.
3. Reduce heat and simmer for about 20 minutes until the sweet potatoes are tender.
4. Use an immersion blender to blend the soup until smooth, or blend in batches in a regular blender.
5. Stir in the coconut milk and heat through.
6. Serve hot.

Nutrition Info per Serving

- Calories: 230
- Protein: 3g
- Fat: 12g
- Carbohydrates: 28g
- Fiber: 5g
- Sugar: 8g

Serves

4

Cooking Time

30 minutes

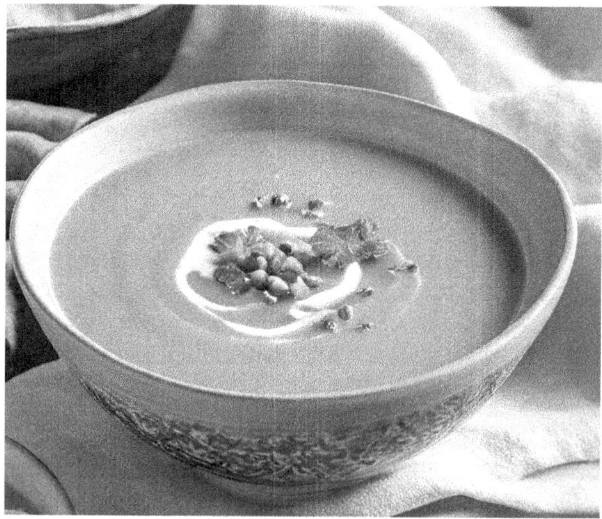

4. Zucchini Noodles with Pesto

Ingredients

- 4 medium zucchinis, spiralized into noodles
- 1 cup fresh basil leaves
- 1/4 cup pine nuts
- 1/4 cup grated Parmesan cheese (optional)
- 2 cloves garlic
- 1/4 cup olive oil
- 1 tablespoon lemon juice

Instructions

1. In a food processor, combine the basil leaves, pine nuts, Parmesan cheese (if using), and garlic. Pulse until finely chopped.
2. With the processor running, slowly add the olive oil and lemon juice until the mixture is smooth.
3. In a large skillet, heat a small amount of olive oil over medium heat. Add the zucchini noodles and cook for about 2-3 minutes until just tender.
4. Remove from heat and toss with the pesto.
5. Serve immediately.

Nutrition Info per Serving

- Calories: 200
- Protein: 4g
- Fat: 18g
- Carbohydrates: 8g
- Fiber: 3g
- Sugar: 4g

Serves

4

Cooking Time

15 minutes

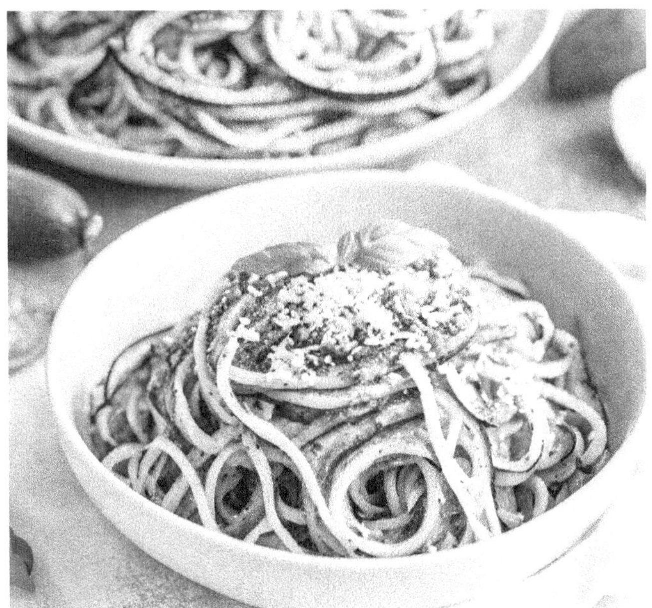

5. Eggplant and Chickpea Stew

Ingredients

- 2 tablespoons olive oil
- 1 onion, finely chopped
- 2 cloves garlic, minced
- 1 large eggplant, diced
- 1 red bell pepper, diced
- 1 can (15 ounces) chickpeas, drained and rinsed
- 1 can (14 ounces) diced tomatoes
- 1 teaspoon ground cumin
- 1 teaspoon ground paprika
- 1 teaspoon dried oregano
- 2 cups vegetable broth

Instructions

1. In a large pot, heat the olive oil over medium heat. Add the onion and garlic, and sauté for about 5 minutes until softened.
2. Add the diced eggplant and red bell pepper, and cook for about 10 minutes until tender.
3. Stir in the chickpeas, diced tomatoes, ground cumin, ground paprika, dried oregano, and vegetable broth. Bring to a boil.
4. Reduce heat and simmer for about 20 minutes until the flavors are well combined.
5. Serve hot.

Nutrition Info per Serving

- Calories: 220
- Protein: 5g
- Fat: 10g
- Carbohydrates: 28g
- Fiber: 8g
- Sugar: 10g

Serves

4

Cooking Time

35 minutes

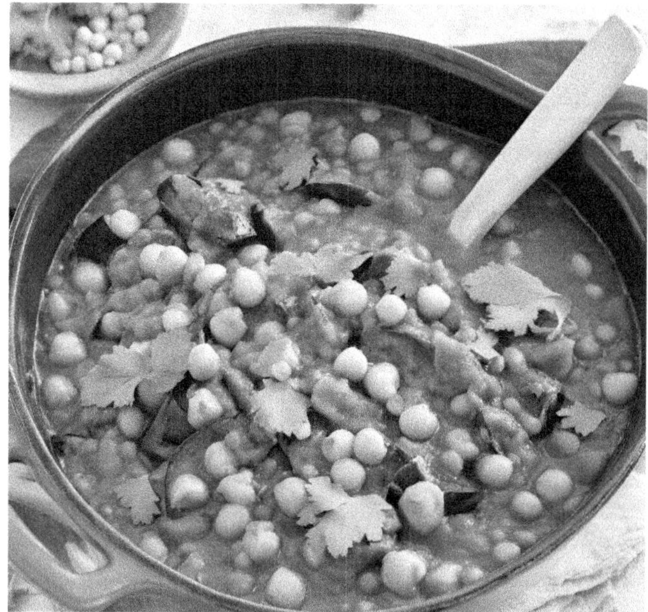

6. Broccoli and Almond Salad

Ingredients

- 4 cups broccoli florets
- 1/2 cup sliced almonds
- 1/4 cup red onion, finely chopped
- 1/4 cup dried cranberries
- 1/4 cup olive oil
- 2 tablespoons apple cider vinegar
- 1 tablespoon honey
- 1 teaspoon Dijon mustard

Instructions

1. Steam the broccoli florets for about 3-4 minutes until tender but still crisp. Allow to cool.
2. In a large bowl, combine the steamed broccoli, sliced almonds, red onion, and dried cranberries.
3. In a small bowl, whisk together the olive oil, apple cider vinegar, honey, and Dijon mustard.
4. Pour the dressing over the broccoli mixture and toss to combine.
5. Serve immediately or refrigerate until ready to serve.

Nutrition Info per Serving

- Calories: 200
- Protein: 4g
- Fat: 16g
- Carbohydrates: 12g
- Fiber: 4g
- Sugar: 7g

Serves
4

Cooking Time
10 minutes

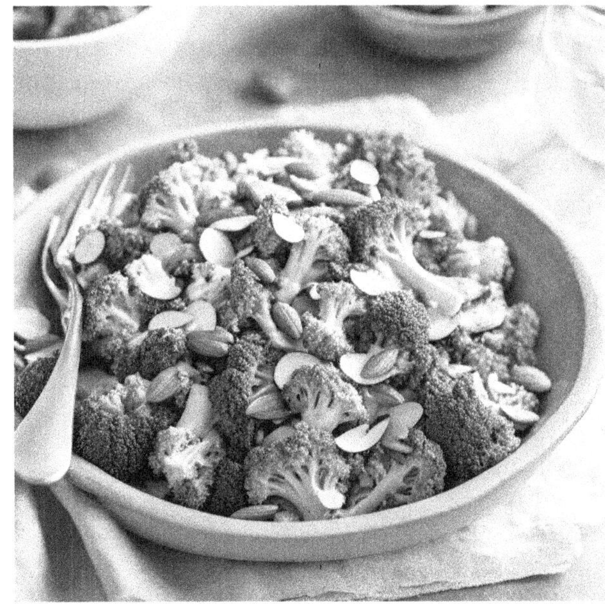

7. Spinach and Mushroom Quiche

Ingredients

- 1 pre-made gluten-free pie crust
- 1 tablespoon olive oil
- 1 onion, finely chopped
- 2 cloves garlic, minced
- 1 cup mushrooms, sliced
- 4 cups fresh spinach, chopped
- 4 large eggs
- 1 cup unsweetened almond milk
- 1/2 cup shredded dairy-free cheese (optional)
- 1 teaspoon dried thyme

Instructions

1. Preheat the oven to 375°F (190°C).
2. In a large skillet, heat the olive oil over medium heat. Add the onion and garlic, and sauté for about 5 minutes until softened.
3. Add the mushrooms and cook for another 5 minutes until they release their juices and are tender.
4. Stir in the chopped spinach and cook until wilted. Remove from heat and let cool slightly.
5. In a large bowl, whisk together the eggs, almond milk, shredded cheese (if using), and dried thyme.
6. Stir the spinach and mushroom mixture into the egg mixture.
7. Pour the filling into the pre-made pie crust.
8. Bake for 35-40 minutes, until the quiche is set and lightly browned on top.
9. Let cool for 10 minutes before slicing and serving.

Nutrition Info per Serving

- Calories: 220
- Protein: 8g
- Fat: 15g
- Carbohydrates: 15g
- Fiber: 3g
- Sugar: 2g

Serves

6

Cooking Time

50 minutes

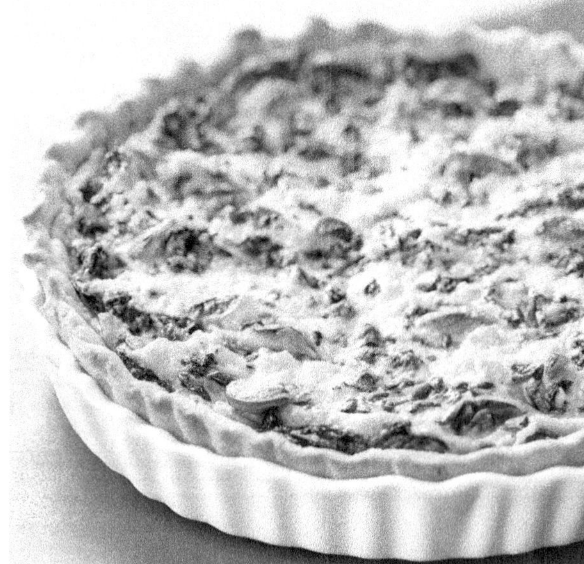

8. Beetroot and Walnut Dip

Ingredients

- 2 large beetroots, roasted and peeled
- 1/2 cup walnuts
- 1/4 cup Greek yogurt
- 1 tablespoon lemon juice
- 2 cloves garlic, minced
- 1 tablespoon olive oil

Instructions

1. Preheat the oven to 400°F (200°C). Wrap the beetroots in foil and roast for about 45-60 minutes until tender. Allow to cool, then peel.
2. In a food processor, combine the roasted beetroots, walnuts, Greek yogurt, lemon juice, minced garlic, and olive oil.
3. Process until smooth and creamy.
4. Serve immediately or chill in the refrigerator until ready to serve.

Nutrition Info per Serving

- Calories: 140
- Protein: 4g
- Fat: 10g
- Carbohydrates: 11g
- Fiber: 3g
- Sugar: 7g

Serves
4
Cooking Time
60 minutes

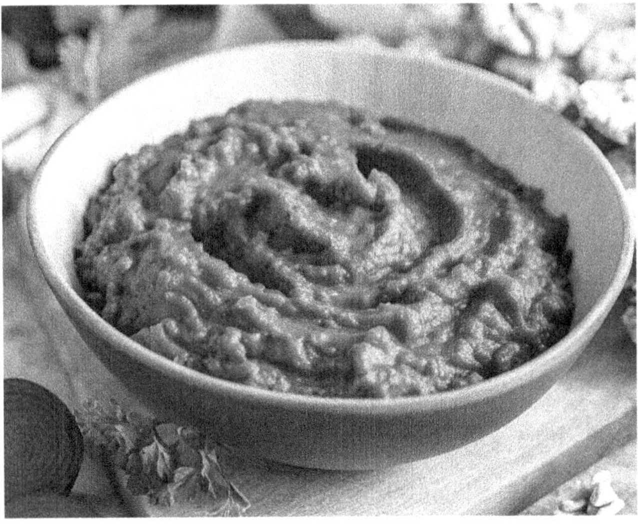

9. Brussels Sprouts with Balsamic Glaze

Ingredients

- 4 cups Brussels sprouts, trimmed and halved
- 2 tablespoons olive oil
- 1/4 cup balsamic vinegar
- 1 tablespoon honey

Instructions

1. Preheat the oven to 400°F (200°C).
2. In a large bowl, toss the Brussels sprouts with olive oil.
3. Spread the Brussels sprouts on a baking sheet in a single layer.
4. Roast for 20-25 minutes, until tender and browned.
5. Meanwhile, in a small saucepan, combine the balsamic vinegar and honey. Simmer over medium heat until the mixture is reduced by half and thickened.
6. Drizzle the balsamic glaze over the roasted Brussels sprouts and toss to coat.
7. Serve immediately.

Nutrition Info per Serving

- Calories: 150
- Protein: 3g
- Fat: 9g
- Carbohydrates: 15g
- Fiber: 4g
- Sugar: 9g

Serves

4

Cooking Time

30 minutes

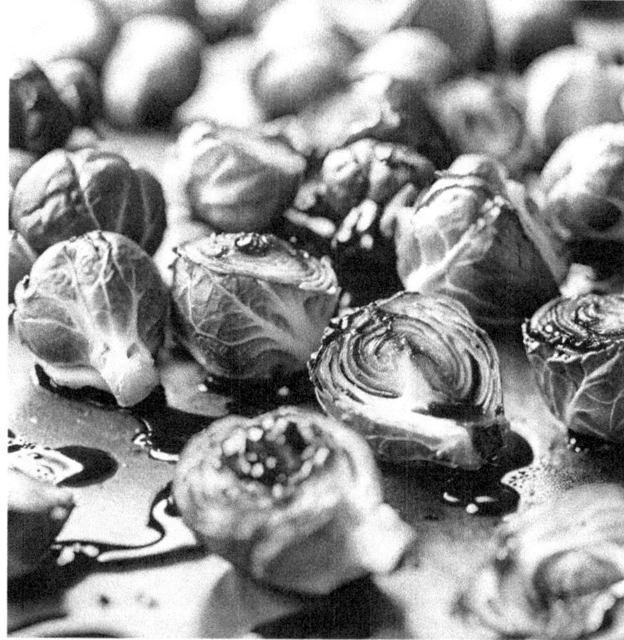

10. Curried Lentil and Vegetable Soup

Ingredients

- 1 tablespoon olive oil
- 1 onion, finely chopped
- 2 cloves garlic, minced
- 1 tablespoon grated fresh ginger
- 1 tablespoon curry powder
- 1 cup dried red lentils
- 4 cups vegetable broth
- 2 carrots, sliced
- 2 celery stalks, sliced
- 1 zucchini, diced
- 1 can (14 ounces) diced tomatoes
- 1 cup coconut milk

Instructions

1. In a large pot, heat the olive oil over medium heat. Add the onion, garlic, and grated ginger, and sauté for about 5 minutes until softened.
2. Stir in the curry powder and cook for 1 minute until fragrant.
3. Add the dried red lentils, vegetable broth, carrots, celery, zucchini, and diced tomatoes. Bring to a boil.
4. Reduce heat and simmer for about 20 minutes until the lentils and vegetables are tender.
5. Stir in the coconut milk and cook for an additional 5 minutes until heated through.
6. Serve hot.

Nutrition Info per Serving

- Calories: 250
- Protein: 10g
- Fat: 10g
- Carbohydrates: 32g
- Fiber: 8g
- Sugar: 8g

Serves

4

Cooking Time

30 minutes

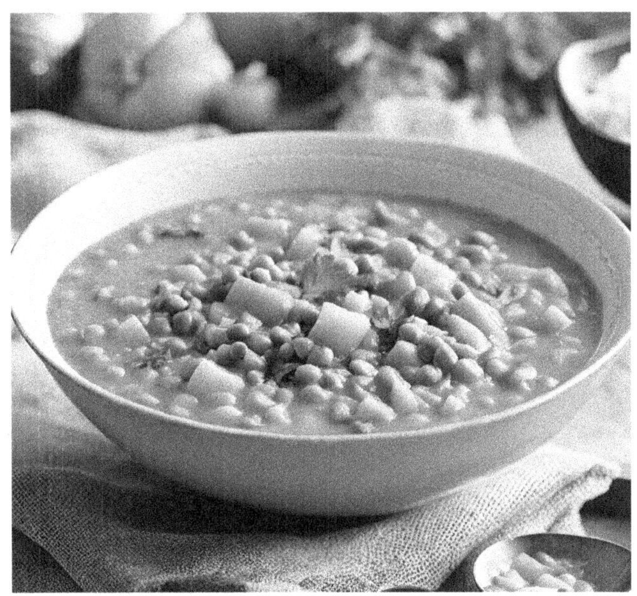

11. Butternut Squash Risotto

Ingredients

- 1 tablespoon olive oil
- 1 onion, finely chopped
- 2 cloves garlic, minced
- 1 1/2 cups Arborio rice
- 4 cups vegetable broth, warmed
- 2 cups butternut squash, peeled and diced
- 1/2 cup white wine (optional)
- 1/4 cup nutritional yeast (optional)
- 1 tablespoon fresh thyme, chopped

Instructions

1. In a large pot, heat the olive oil over medium heat. Add the onion and garlic, and sauté for about 5 minutes until softened.
2. Stir in the Arborio rice and cook for about 2 minutes until the rice is lightly toasted.
3. Add the white wine (if using) and cook until it is mostly absorbed.
4. Add the diced butternut squash and 1 cup of the warmed vegetable broth. Cook, stirring frequently, until the liquid is absorbed.
5. Continue to add the broth, 1 cup at a time, stirring frequently and allowing the liquid to be absorbed before adding more, until the rice is creamy and the butternut squash is tender, about 20 minutes.
6. Stir in the nutritional yeast (if using) and fresh thyme.
7. Serve hot.

Nutrition Info per Serving

- Calories: 320
- Protein: 7g
- Fat: 6g
- Carbohydrates: 59g
- Fiber: 4g
- Sugar: 4g

Serves

4

Cooking Time

30 minutes

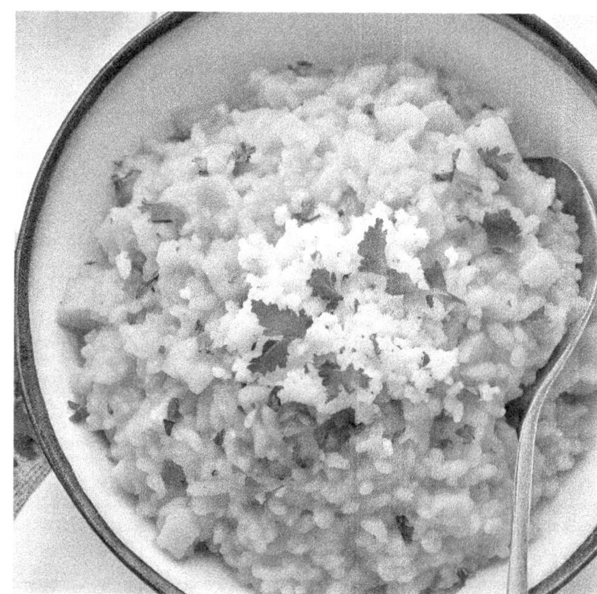

12. Vegetable Stir-Fry with Tofu

Ingredients

- 1 tablespoon coconut oil
- 1 block firm tofu, pressed and cubed
- 1 onion, sliced
- 2 cloves garlic, minced
- 1 red bell pepper, sliced
- 1 yellow bell pepper, sliced
- 1 cup broccoli florets
- 1 carrot, julienned
- 1/4 cup tamari (gluten-free soy sauce)
- 1 tablespoon sesame oil
- 1 tablespoon sesame seeds
- 1 tablespoon fresh ginger, grated

Instructions

1. In a large skillet or wok, heat the coconut oil over medium-high heat.
2. Add the cubed tofu and cook for about 5-7 minutes until golden brown. Remove from the skillet and set aside.
3. In the same skillet, add the onion, garlic, and fresh ginger. Cook for about 2 minutes until fragrant.
4. Add the red and yellow bell peppers, broccoli florets, and carrot. Stir-fry for about 5-7 minutes until the vegetables are tender-crisp.
5. Return the tofu to the skillet and stir in the tamari and sesame oil. Cook for an additional 2 minutes until heated through.
6. Sprinkle with sesame seeds and serve hot.

Nutrition Info per Serving

- Calories: 250
- Protein: 15g
- Fat: 15g
- Carbohydrates: 15g
- Fiber: 5g
- Sugar: 5g

Serves

4

Cooking Time

20 minutes

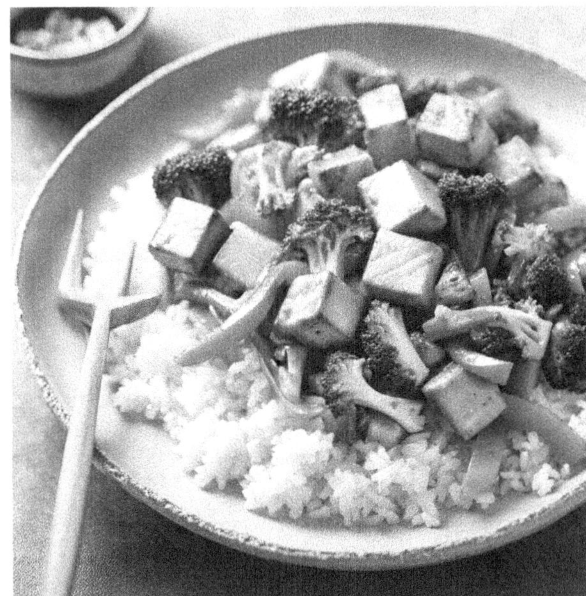

13. Cabbage Slaw with Sesame Dressing

Ingredients

- 4 cups green cabbage, shredded
- 2 cups red cabbage, shredded
- 1 cup carrots, julienned
- 1/4 cup green onions, chopped
- 2 tablespoons sesame seeds
- 1/4 cup rice vinegar
- 2 tablespoons tamari (gluten-free soy sauce)
- 1 tablespoon honey
- 1 tablespoon sesame oil
- 1 teaspoon fresh ginger, grated

Instructions

1. In a large bowl, combine the shredded green and red cabbage, julienned carrots, and chopped green onions.
2. In a small bowl, whisk together the rice vinegar, tamari, honey, sesame oil, and fresh ginger.
3. Pour the dressing over the cabbage mixture and toss to coat evenly.
4. Sprinkle with sesame seeds.
5. Serve immediately or refrigerate until ready to serve.

Nutrition Info per Serving

- Calories: 100
- Protein: 2g
- Fat: 5g
- Carbohydrates: 12g
- Fiber: 3g
- Sugar: 7g

Serves

4

Cooking Time

15 minutes

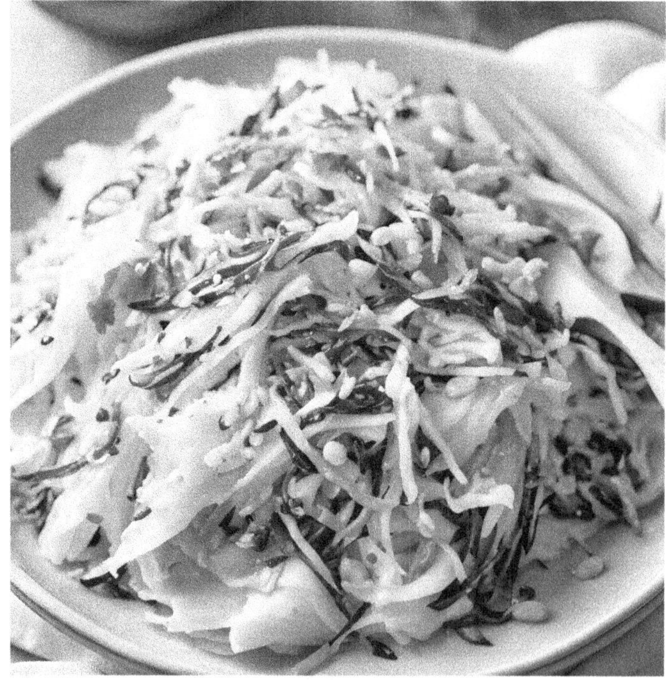

14. Portobello Mushroom Caps with Quinoa

Ingredients

- 4 large Portobello mushroom caps
- 1 cup quinoa, rinsed
- 2 cups vegetable broth
- 1 onion, finely chopped
- 2 cloves garlic, minced
- 1 cup spinach, chopped
- 1/4 cup sun-dried tomatoes, chopped
- 1/4 cup pine nuts, toasted
- 1 tablespoon olive oil

Instructions

1. Preheat the oven to 375°F (190°C).
2. In a medium saucepan, bring the vegetable broth to a boil. Add the quinoa, reduce heat to low, cover, and simmer for 15 minutes until the quinoa is tender and the broth is absorbed. Set aside.
3. In a skillet, heat the olive oil over medium heat. Add the onion and garlic, and sauté for about 5 minutes until softened.
4. Stir in the chopped spinach and sun-dried tomatoes, and cook until the spinach is wilted.
5. Remove from heat and stir in the cooked quinoa and toasted pine nuts.
6. Place the Portobello mushroom caps on a baking sheet and spoon the quinoa mixture into each cap.
7. Bake for 20 minutes until the mushrooms are tender.
8. Serve hot.

Nutrition Info per Serving

- Calories: 220
- Protein: 8g
- Fat: 10g
- Carbohydrates: 26g
- Fiber: 5g
- Sugar: 5g

Serves

4

Cooking Time

30 minutes

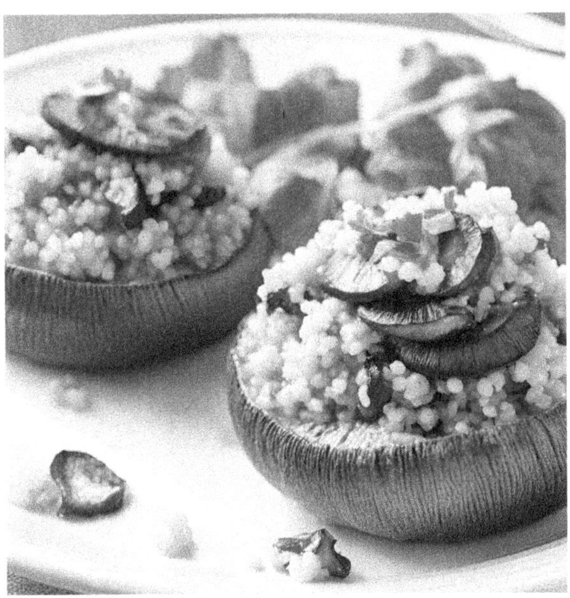

15. Spaghetti Squash with Tomato Sauce

Ingredients

- 1 large spaghetti squash
- 1 tablespoon olive oil
- 1 onion, finely chopped
- 2 cloves garlic, minced
- 1 can (14 ounces) diced tomatoes
- 1 teaspoon dried basil
- 1 teaspoon dried oregano
- 1/4 cup fresh basil, chopped (optional)

Instructions

1. Preheat the oven to 375°F (190°C). Cut the spaghetti squash in half lengthwise and scoop out the seeds.
2. Place the squash halves cut-side down on a baking sheet and roast for 35-40 minutes until tender. Allow to cool slightly, then use a fork to scrape out the spaghetti-like strands.
3. While the squash is roasting, heat the olive oil in a skillet over medium heat. Add the onion and garlic, and sauté for about 5 minutes until softened.
4. Stir in the diced tomatoes, dried basil, and dried oregano. Simmer for about 10 minutes until the sauce thickens.
5. Serve the roasted spaghetti squash topped with the tomato sauce and fresh basil if using.

Nutrition Info per Serving

- Calories: 150
- Protein: 3g
- Fat: 7g
- Carbohydrates: 20g
- Fiber: 4g
- Sugar: 8g

Serves

4

Cooking Time

45 minutes

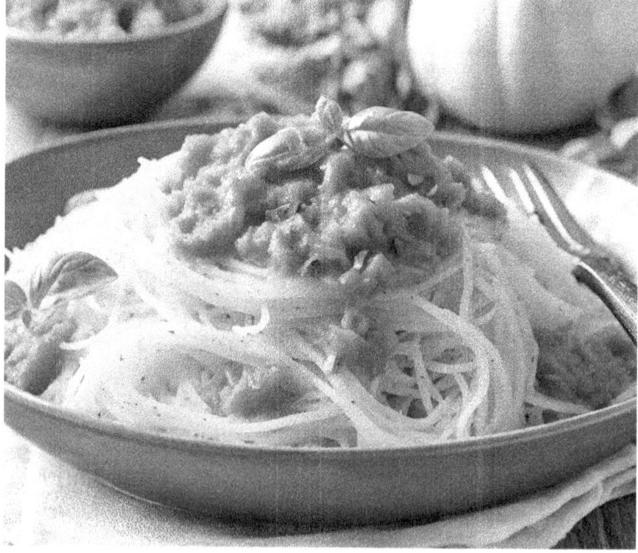

10-WEEK MEAL PLAN

Week 1
Day 1
- Breakfast: Flaxseed and Banana Muffins
- Lunch: Broccoli and Almond Salad
- Dinner: Grilled Salmon with Dill Sauce and steamed asparagus

Day 2
- Breakfast: Polenta with Grilled Vegetables
- Lunch: Turkey and Cranberry Salad
- Dinner: Butternut Squash Risotto

Day 3
- Breakfast: Kefir with Chopped Dates
- Lunch: Chicken and Mango Chutney Sandwiches
- Dinner: Eggplant and Chickpea Stew

Day 4
- Breakfast: Apple Cinnamon Baked Oatmeal
- Lunch: Spinach and Mushroom Quiche
- Dinner: Turkey Soup with Kale and White Beans

Day 5
- Breakfast: Savory Spinach Pancakes
- Lunch: Cabbage Slaw with Sesame Dressing
- Dinner: Chicken Ginger Soup

Day 6
- Breakfast: Nutty Porridge
- Lunch: Portobello Mushroom Caps with Quinoa
- Dinner: Lemon Herb Roasted Chicken

Day 7
- Breakfast: Berry and Kiwi Salad
- Lunch: Spaghetti Squash with Tomato Sauce
- Dinner: Herb Roasted Turkey Thighs

Week 2
Day 8
- Breakfast: Raspberry Coconut Porridge
- Lunch: Grilled Trout with Almondine Sauce and steamed broccoli
- Dinner: Cauliflower and Hemp Seed Soup

Day 9

- Breakfast: Overnight Hemp Seeds
- Lunch: Sweet Potato and Ginger Soup
- Dinner: Chicken and Asparagus Stir-Fry

Day 10

- Breakfast: Tempeh Bacon Lettuce Tomato Sandwich
- Lunch: Zucchini Noodles with Pesto
- Dinner: Smoky Turkey Chili

Day 11

- Breakfast: Oatmeal with Berries
- Lunch: Beetroot and Walnut Dip with vegetable sticks
- Dinner: Curried Lentil and Vegetable Soup

Day 12

- Breakfast: Almond Yogurt with Honey and Walnuts
- Lunch: Balsamic Glazed Turkey Breast with mixed greens
- Dinner: Chicken Ratatouille

Day 13

- Breakfast: Quinoa Breakfast Bowl
- Lunch: Grilled Chicken with Avocado Salsa
- Dinner: Vegetable Stir-Fry with Tofu

Day 14

- Breakfast: Turmeric Porridge
- Lunch: Brussels Sprouts with Balsamic Glaze
- Dinner: Stuffed Turkey Breast with Spinach and Walnuts

Week 3

Day 15

- Breakfast: Buckwheat Pancakes
- Lunch: Apple and Parsnip Soup
- Dinner: Garlic and Lemon Roasted Chicken Thighs

Day 16

- Breakfast: Fruit and Nut Platter
- Lunch: Roasted Red Pepper Soup
- Dinner: Turkey Veggie Meatloaf

Day 17

- Breakfast: Flaxseed and Banana Muffins
- Lunch: Cabbage Slaw with Sesame Dressing
- Dinner: Grilled Salmon with Dill Sauce and steamed green beans

Day 18
- Breakfast: Polenta with Grilled Vegetables
- Lunch: Turkey and Cranberry Salad
- Dinner: Fish Curry with Coconut Milk

Day 19
- Breakfast: Kefir with Chopped Dates
- Lunch: Spinach and Mushroom Quiche
- Dinner: Chicken Zoodle Soup

Day 20
- Breakfast: Apple Cinnamon Baked Oatmeal
- Lunch: Portobello Mushroom Caps with Quinoa
- Dinner: Smoky Turkey Chili

Day 21
- Breakfast: Savory Spinach Pancakes
- Lunch: Beetroot and Walnut Dip with gluten-free crackers
- Dinner: Lemon Herb Roasted Chicken

Week 4

Day 22
- Breakfast: Nutty Porridge
- Lunch: Spaghetti Squash with Tomato Sauce
- Dinner: Grilled Trout with Almondine Sauce and roasted Brussels sprouts

Day 23
- Breakfast: Berry and Kiwi Salad
- Lunch: Curried Lentil and Vegetable Soup
- Dinner: Chicken Ginger Soup

Day 24
- Breakfast: Raspberry Coconut Porridge
- Lunch: Cabbage Slaw with Sesame Dressing
- Dinner: Stuffed Turkey Breast with Spinach and Walnuts

Day 25
- Breakfast: Overnight Hemp Seeds
- Lunch: Balsamic Glazed Turkey Breast with mixed greens
- Dinner: Chicken and Broccoli Alfredo

Day 26
- Breakfast: Tempeh Bacon Lettuce Tomato Sandwich
- Lunch: Sweet Potato and Ginger Soup
- Dinner: Eggplant and Chickpea Stew

Day 27
- Breakfast: Oatmeal with Berries
- Lunch: Grilled Chicken with Avocado Salsa
- Dinner: Vegetable Stir-Fry with Tofu

Day 28
- Breakfast: Almond Yogurt with Honey and Walnuts
- Lunch: Zucchini Noodles with Pesto
- Dinner: Garlic and Lemon Roasted Chicken Thighs

Week 5

Day 29
- Breakfast: Quinoa Breakfast Bowl
- Lunch: Apple and Parsnip Soup
- Dinner: Chicken Ratatouille

Day 30
- Breakfast: Turmeric Porridge
- Lunch: Roasted Red Pepper Soup
- Dinner: Turkey Veggie Meatloaf

Day 31
- Breakfast: Buckwheat Pancakes
- Lunch: Brussels Sprouts with Balsamic Glaze
- Dinner: Fish Curry with Coconut Milk

Day 32
- Breakfast: Fruit and Nut Platter
- Lunch: Spinach and Mushroom Quiche
- Dinner: Chicken Zoodle Soup

Day 33
- Breakfast: Flaxseed and Banana Muffins
- Lunch: Beetroot and Walnut Dip with vegetable sticks
- Dinner: Smoky Turkey Chili

Day 34
- Breakfast: Polenta with Grilled Vegetables
- Lunch: Portobello Mushroom Caps with Quinoa
- Dinner: Grilled Salmon with Dill Sauce and steamed green beans

Day 35
- Breakfast: Kefir with Chopped Dates
- Lunch: Turkey and Cranberry Salad
- Dinner: Lemon Herb Roasted Chicken

Week 6

Day 36
- Breakfast: Flaxseed and Banana Muffins
- Lunch: Watercress Soup
- Dinner: Herb-Crusted Cod with steamed green beans

Day 37
- Breakfast: Savory Spinach Pancakes
- Lunch: Vegan Mushroom Stroganoff Soup
- Dinner: Chicken and Spinach Stew

Day 38
- Breakfast: Nutty Porridge
- Lunch: Grilled Salmon with Avocado Salsa
- Dinner: Squash and Apple Stew

Day 39
- Breakfast: Raspberry Coconut Porridge
- Lunch: Celery Root and Apple Soup
- Dinner: Chicken and Asparagus Stir-Fry

Day 40
- Breakfast: Overnight Hemp Seeds
- Lunch: Caribbean Chickpea and Potato Curry
- Dinner: Garlic Butter Halibut with roasted Brussels sprouts

Day 41
- Breakfast: Tempeh Bacon Lettuce Tomato Sandwich
- Lunch: Turkey and Cranberry Salad
- Dinner: Spaghetti Squash with Tomato Sauce

Day 42
- Breakfast: Oatmeal with Berries
- Lunch: Chicken and Mango Chutney Sandwiches
- Dinner: Fish Stew with Tomatoes

Week 7

Day 43
- Breakfast: Almond Yogurt with Honey and Walnuts
- Lunch: Kale and Quinoa Salad
- Dinner: Cauliflower and Hemp Seed Soup

Day 44
- Breakfast: Quinoa Breakfast Bowl
- Lunch: Curried Lentil and Vegetable Soup
- Dinner: Mediterranean Turkey Meatloaf

Day 45
- Breakfast: Turmeric Porridge
- Lunch: Brussels Sprouts with Balsamic Glaze
- Dinner: Chicken and Broccoli Alfredo

Day 46
- Breakfast: Buckwheat Pancakes
- Lunch: Eggplant and Chickpea Stew
- Dinner: Smoky Turkey Chili

Day 47
- Breakfast: Fruit and Nut Platter
- Lunch: Chicken Ginger Soup
- Dinner: Grilled Trout with Almondine Sauce and steamed broccoli

Day 48
- Breakfast: Polenta with Grilled Vegetables
- Lunch: Spinach and Mushroom Quiche
- Dinner: Turkey Stuffed Peppers

Day 49
- Breakfast: Kefir with Chopped Dates
- Lunch: Beetroot and Walnut Dip with vegetable sticks
- Dinner: Lemon Garlic Shrimp Pasta

Week 8

Day 50
- Breakfast: Apple Cinnamon Baked Oatmeal
- Lunch: Balsamic Glazed Turkey Breast with mixed greens
- Dinner: Chicken Zoodle Soup

Day 51
- Breakfast: Savory Spinach Pancakes
- Lunch: Turkey Soup with Kale and White Beans
- Dinner: Garlic and Lemon Roasted Chicken Thighs

Day 52
- Breakfast: Nutty Porridge
- Lunch: Zucchini Noodles with Pesto
- Dinner: Herb Roasted Turkey Thighs

Day 53
- Breakfast: Berry and Kiwi Salad
- Lunch: Cabbage Slaw with Sesame Dressing
- Dinner: Chicken Ratatouille

Day 54
- Breakfast: Raspberry Coconut Porridge
- Lunch: Portobello Mushroom Caps with Quinoa
- Dinner: Peppered Tuna Steak with roasted Brussels sprouts

Day 55
- Breakfast: Overnight Hemp Seeds
- Lunch: Sweet Potato and Ginger Soup
- Dinner: Turkey Veggie Meatloaf

Day 56
- Breakfast: Tempeh Bacon Lettuce Tomato Sandwich
- Lunch: Spaghetti Squash with Tomato Sauce
- Dinner: Shrimp and Broccoli Alfredo

Week 9

Day 57
- Breakfast: Oatmeal with Berries
- Lunch: Vegan Mushroom Stroganoff Soup
- Dinner: Grilled Salmon with Dill Sauce and steamed asparagus

Day 58
- Breakfast: Almond Yogurt with Honey and Walnuts
- Lunch: Celery Root and Apple Soup
- Dinner: Chicken and Spinach Stew

Day 59
- Breakfast: Quinoa Breakfast Bowl
- Lunch: Curried Lentil and Vegetable Soup
- Dinner: Fish Stew with Tomatoes

Day 60
- Breakfast: Turmeric Porridge
- Lunch: Kale and Quinoa Salad
- Dinner: Herb-Crusted Cod with roasted Brussels sprouts

Day 61
- Breakfast: Buckwheat Pancakes
- Lunch: Chicken and Mango Chutney Sandwiches
- Dinner: Stuffed Turkey Breast with Spinach and Walnuts

Day 62
- Breakfast: Fruit and Nut Platter
- Lunch: Turkey and Cranberry Salad
- Dinner: Butternut Squash Risotto

Day 63
- Breakfast: Polenta with Grilled Vegetables
- Lunch: Brussels Sprouts with Balsamic Glaze
- Dinner: Lemon Garlic Shrimp Pasta

Week 10

Day 64

- Breakfast: Kefir with Chopped Dates
- Lunch: Watercress Soup
- Dinner: Chicken and Asparagus Stir-Fry

Day 65

- Breakfast: Apple Cinnamon Baked Oatmeal
- Lunch: Spinach and Mushroom Quiche
- Dinner: Grilled Trout with Almondine Sauce and steamed green beans

Day 66

- Breakfast: Savory Spinach Pancakes
- Lunch: Beetroot and Walnut Dip with gluten-free crackers
- Dinner: Cauliflower and Hemp Seed Soup

Day 67

- Breakfast: Nutty Porridge
- Lunch: Eggplant and Chickpea Stew
- Dinner: Herb Roasted Turkey Thighs

Day 68

- Breakfast: Berry and Kiwi Salad
- Lunch: Cabbage Slaw with Sesame Dressing
- Dinner: Chicken Ratatouille

Day 69

- Breakfast: Raspberry Coconut Porridge
- Lunch: Turkey Soup with Kale and White Beans
- Dinner: Garlic Butter Halibut with roasted Brussels sprouts

Day 70

- Breakfast: Overnight Hemp Seeds
- Lunch: Portobello Mushroom Caps with Quinoa
- Dinner: Smoky Turkey Chili

Weekly Meal planner+ Journal

	BREAKFAST	LUNCH	DINNER	SNACKS
MON				
TUE				
WED				
THU				
FRI				
SAT				
SUN				

What are your specific goals for following the Lichen Sclerosus diet? How do you hope it will improve your symptoms or overall health?

....

....

....

....

....

....

Weekly Meal planner+ Journal

	BREAKFAST	LUNCH	DINNER	SNACKS
MON				
TUE				
WED				
THU				
FRI				
SAT				
SUN				

Describe your current eating habits. What foods do you eat regularly, and which ones do you think you should avoid?

....

....

....

....

....

....

Weekly Meal planner + Journal

	BREAKFAST	LUNCH	DINNER	SNACKS
MON				
TUE				
WED				
THU				
FRI				
SAT				
SUN				

What changes will you need to make to your grocery shopping list to align with the Lichen Sclerosus diet? Are there any new foods you will need to add?

Weekly Meal planner+ Journal

	BREAKFAST	LUNCH	DINNER	SNACKS
MON				
TUE				
WED				
THU				
FRI				
SAT				
SUN				

What are some new recipes you are excited to try that fit within the Lichen Sclerosus diet guidelines?

....

....

....

....

....

....

Weekly Meal planner+ Journal

	BREAKFAST	LUNCH	DINNER	SNACKS
MON				
TUE				
WED				
THU				
FRI				
SAT				
SUN				

How can you make healthier choices when eating out at restaurants? What are some strategies to avoid foods that might trigger your symptoms?

....

....

....

....

....

....

Weekly Meal planner+ Journal

	BREAKFAST	LUNCH	DINNER	SNACKS
MON				
TUE				
WED				
THU				
FRI				
SAT				
SUN				

Keep a food diary for one week. Record everything you eat and any symptoms you experience. Are there any patterns or specific foods that seem to trigger your symptoms?

Weekly Meal planner+ Journal

	BREAKFAST	LUNCH	DINNER	SNACKS
MON				
TUE				
WED				
THU				
FRI				
SAT				
SUN				

Who can you rely on for support as you transition to the Lichen Sclerosus diet? How can they help you stay accountable and motivated?

....

....

....

....

....

....

....

Weekly Meal planner+ Journal

	BREAKFAST	LUNCH	DINNER	SNACKS
MON				
TUE				
WED				
THU				
FRI				
SAT				
SUN				

What challenges do you anticipate facing while following the Lichen Sclerosus diet? How can you prepare to overcome these challenges?

....

....

....

....

....

....

Weekly Meal planner+ Journal

	BREAKFAST	LUNCH	DINNER	SNACKS
MON				
TUE				
WED				
THU				
FRI				
SAT				
SUN				

What positive changes have you noticed since starting the Lichen Sclerosus diet? How do these changes motivate you to continue?

....

....

....

....

....

....

Weekly Meal planner+ Journal

	BREAKFAST	LUNCH	DINNER	SNACKS
MON				
TUE				
WED				
THU				
FRI				
SAT				
SUN				

What are your long-term health goals related to managing Lichen Sclerosus? How can the diet help you achieve these goals?

....

....

....

....

....

....

Weekly Meal planner+ Journal

	BREAKFAST	LUNCH	DINNER	SNACKS
MON				
TUE				
WED				
THU				
FRI				
SAT				
SUN				

After following the Lichen Sclerosus diet for a month, reflect on your journey. What has been the most significant change for you, and what have you learned about your body and your health?

....

....

....

....

....

....

Scan the QR code below to get a surprise bonus